What the experts are saying:

"This is a very important and readable book, with broader implications than the title implies. For women who are fortunate enough to be properly fitted and trained, the cervical cap may be the nearest thing to an ideal contraceptive that exists today. It is free of serious side effects, inexpensive and, unlike other 'barriers,' disassociated from the act of love. Ms. Chalker, a longtime provider, is one of the foremost experts on the cap, a careful scholar and a lucid writer as well. I hope that every woman who is tired of risking her health for the sake of her sexuality will read this book."

—Barbara Seaman
Coauthor with Gideon Seaman, M.D., of
Women and the Crisis in Sex Hormones
and author of *Free and Female*

"The revival of the cervical cap is an exciting event for women, and *The Complete Cervical Cap Guide* illuminates every aspect of its use—past, present and future."
—Shere Hite

"Comprehensive and meticulously researched, *The Complete Cervical Cap* [Guide] sets a new standard for informational books on birth control and offers a splendid blend of policy and how-to advice that will be equally appealing to doctors, health educators, and women seeking an alternative method of birth control."

—Gary Richwald, M.D.
Division of Population and Family Health
UCLA School of Public Health

Cap users rave about this birth control option:

"The cap is great. I've used every birth control method except sterilization, so I should know."—*Atlanta, Ga.*

"I love the cap because you need so little spermicide and can have sex with more frequency."—*New York, N.Y.*

"The cervical cap is so comfortable it makes the diaphragm seem like a Frisbee."—*Oakland, Calif.*

"It's truly spontaneous and I don't get chronic bladder infections like I did from the diaphragm."—*New Brunswick, N.J.*

"The cap is small and efficient. It works without affecting your whole body like the Pill."—*New York, N.Y.*

"I've used the cap for three years and have never used anything else. Right now, I don't want to. . . . This is so great!"
—*Boston, Mass.*

✻ ✻ ✻ ✻ ✻ ✻ ✻ ✻ ✻ ✻ ✻

THE COMPLETE CERVICAL CAP GUIDE

REBECCA CHALKER

Illustrated by Suzann Gage

1817

Harper & Row, Publishers, New York

Cambridge, Philadelphia, San Francisco, Washington
London, Mexico City, São Paulo, Singapore, Sydney

✻ ✻ ✻ ✻ ✻ ✻ ✻ ✻ ✻ ✻ ✻

To the modern cervical cap pioneers
in the United States
who looked into the past
and discovered the future

FIRST EDITION

Designer: Ruth Bornschlegel

Copy Editor: Rick Hermann

Index: Maro Riofrancos

Library of Congress Cataloging-in-Publication Data

Chalker, Rebecca.
  The complete cervical cap guide.
  Bibliography: p.

  Includes index.
  1. Cervical caps. I. Title.
RG137.2.C47   1987   613.9'435   86-45646
ISBN 0-06-055068-6   87 88 89 90 91 MPC 8 7 6 5 4 3 2 1
ISBN 0-06-096113-9 (pbk) 87 88 89 90 91 MPC 8 7 6 5 4 3 2 1

CONTENTS

FOREWORD

During the past fifty years, obstetricians and gynecologists have witnessed tremendous progress in legislation and public attitudes concerning contraception. In the past, scientific medical journals rarely published articles dealing with pregnancy prevention; now, there is a flood of papers on mechanical and hormonal methods of birth control. Once labeled an "obscene" practice by the 1873 Comstock Act, contraception has now become an integral part of obstetrics and gynecology and is included in medical curricula. These drastic changes have produced a pronounced decrease in illness and death connected with pregnancy and childbirth and have provided the tools to plan pregnancies.

This progress was largely due to the pioneering work of courageous American feminists, the foremost of whom were Emma Goldman and Margaret Sanger, who were both imprisoned for advocating birth control. It is partly due to feminist influence that research in contraception has centered more on female methods, placing contraception under the control of women.

In 1954, Margaret Sanger wrote to me referring to an article on the cervical cap which I had co-authored with Drs. Christopher Tietze and George Liebmann:

> I am very much interested in your reprint on the use of the cervical cap. This, as you doubtless know was

the first mechanical device that I brought over from France, back as far as 1912 or 1913, when I went over to study the French method. It was also, by the way, that little cap that used to be shipped to American purchasers under the guise of bonbons from France, and caused Comstock to appear before Congress and receive the congressional privilege of opening packages that came in from Europe through the U.S. mails. After some floundering around trying to get information I found the Ware Company of Philadelphia able to manufacture a cervical cap, and avoided the Federal law by making it in two parts, the cap to be stretched over the rim. This was in use a very long time, and in some parts of the country, where the diaphram is unknown [the cap] is still in use . . . Marie Stopes did not like the Dutch diaphragm and had the cervical cap manufactured in England, calling it by her own invented name, I have forgotten just what.* But she probably had more experience with the use of the cervical cap than any other clinical company.†

In the United States, the use of barrier methods, both male and female, has recently increased, due in part to the virtual disappearance of the IUD from the market. This narrowing of available contraceptive choices puts American women into a difficult situation. The reluctance of U.S. companies to expose themselves to medically unfounded law suits is in large part responsible for this crisis in contraception. In addition, the fear of sexually transmitted diseases has prompted renewed interest in barrier methods. It is an accepted medical fact that barrier methods provide a high degree of protection against sexually transmitted diseases, especially genital herpes, AIDS, and Chlamydia.

The available barrier methods, such as the condom and the diaphragm, are effective but unacceptable to a number of users. The cervical cap, invented in 1838 by Friedrich A. Wilde, a German physician, has a long and interesting history

---

* The name of Marie Stopes's cap is "Prorace." This device is similar and possibly identical to the Prentif rubber cap.

† Personal letter from Margaret Sanger, June 14, 1954. Used by permission of Dr. Grant Sanger.

and is still widely used in Europe. It was also available in the United States until domestic companies stopped its production and practitioners became dependent on caps of foreign manufacture. In 1980, Lamberts, Ltd., an English company, was licensed to supply the Prentif cap to a limited number of U.S. practitioners approved by the Food and Drug Administration (FDA) to provide it on an "investigational basis." Approval of the Prentif cap should offer American women an additional birth control option.

The favorable results of the clinical investigations conducted on the Prentif rubber cap should promote research on other cervical cap models. It is hoped that official endorsement will soon be extended to caps made of lucite and other inert materials which were manufactured and sold in the United States in the past. They appear to be superior in performance and acceptability and, in contrast to the rubber device, can be left in place from menstruation to menstruation, providing prolonged protection.

At the 12th World Congress of Fertility and Sterility in Singapore in October 1986, Dr. Malcolm Potts described the United States as "an underdeveloped country in terms of family planning." It seems senseless for such a resourceful country as the United States to fall into this category. If this crisis is to be resolved, more rather than fewer birth control options must be available. Official sanction of the cervical cap as an alternative barrier method would certainly help in the solution of this crisis.

Hans Lehfeldt, M.D.
Clinical Professor
Department of Obstetrics and Gynecology
New York University School of Medicine

ACKNOWLEDGMENTS

Many, many people contributed to the ideas and material that have come to be called *The Complete Cervical Cap Guide*.

Carol Downer suggested that I write a book on the cap in 1981.

My co-workers in the Federation of Feminist Women's Health Centers taught me to fit cervical caps and afforded me ample experience in their provision. The Chico Feminist Women's Health Center supported the founding of Womancap in New York City. Lynn Thogersen of the Atlanta Feminist Women's Health Center spent many hours talking to me about caps.

I wish to thank my editor at Harper & Row, Janet Goldstein, whose vision made this book possible, whose sensibilities informed its contents throughout, and whose unwavering moral support helped me through some very hard times. I would also like to thank Harper & Row production editor Daril Bentley for his contributions through the production process.

Many cervical cap investigators generously shared their time with me in person and on the phone, and answered a questionnaire about their experiences with the cap.

Several librarians helped me track down essential materials: Gloria Roberts and Zeau Modig at Planned Parenthood's Katherine Douglas McCormick Library; Jean Swinton, librarian at the offices of the New York City Planned Parenthood; Susan Tew of the Alan Guttmacher Institute; Arthur James of the Population Council; and Dolan Willman of the University of Colorado at Denver.

Barbara Seaman, Carol Downer, Gary Richwald, M.D., and Robert A. Hatcher, M.D., gave critical readings of the draft manuscript, and Barbara Feldman read the section on fertility awareness.

Lynn Keresy of the Los Angeles Cervical Cap Study provided me with certain information that was difficult to obtain.

Dr. James Reed, Dean of the History Department at Rutgers University, supplied me with a copy of Emma Goldman's pamphlet of birth control advice.

Dr. Lillian Yin, Director of the Office of Device Evaluation of the Food and Drug Administration and Dr. D. J. Patanelli of the Center of Population Research of the National Institute of Child Health and Human Development generously answered my endless questions about federal policy and procedures.

Many women and men answered a user questionnaire and telephone calls about their experiences with the cervical cap.

Finally, this book could not have been written without encouragement from my co-workers at Ballantine Books, especially Beth Davey and Beverly Robinson, whose understanding about my "other job" made life bearable.

THE COMPLETE CERVICAL CAP GUIDE

1 ✳ JUST ANOTHER MIRACLE DEVICE?
Myths and Realities of the
Cervical Cap

If the diaphragm is regarded as the Queen of birth control, the cap might be called the Anastasia, or lost Princess.
—Barbara Seaman and Gideon Seaman, M.D.
Women and the Crisis in Sex Hormones

The existence of the cervical cap is surely one of the best-kept secrets of the twentieth century. In looking back, it's hard to believe that such a serviceable birth control device, which is as safe and effective as the diaphragm and yet has some of the convenience of the Pill and IUD, got lost.

Naturally, people wonder what happened to the cap, what —or who—prompted its sudden return, and why approval by the Food and Drug Administration (FDA) took so long. If you are a prospective cervical cap user, you probably wonder why an antique barrier method is suddenly being touted as a long-awaited "miracle device." If you are a satisfied diaphragm user, or have at least adjusted to its eccentricities, you will no doubt wonder if the cap is going to be significantly better. If you are a doctor or nurse, you might ask why you never heard about the cap in school or read about it in professional journals.

The Complete Cervical Cap Guide will answer these specific questions and many others about the cap's history and renaissance in North America and its use and effectiveness. The *Guide* also examines the current contraceptive crisis and takes a look at the impact this intriguing device is likely to have.

WHAT IS THE CERVICAL CAP?

Roughly half a dozen cervical cap designs are manufactured today—down from perhaps fifty in Europe during the 1920s and 1930s—but only the Prentif cavity rim cervical cap, made by Lamberts Ltd. of London, is being approved by the FDA for general use in the United States. It is possible that approval of a second cap made by Lamberts, the Dumas, will follow the Prentif within a year or two.

The Prentif cervical cap looks like a large rubber thimble with a soft latex dome and a firm but pliant rim. With a dollop of spermicide placed in the dome, the cap rim is folded in half, tipped into the opening of the vagina, and guided with a finger to the back of the vaginal canal where it readily slips over the cervix (the neck of the uterus). The cap stays firmly in place by gripping the cervix and forming a strong suction, and provides a physical barrier to the sperm, while the spermicide affords an additional chemical barrier.

Because it is smaller and more compact than the diaphragm, the Prentif has several distinct advantages. There is no large spring rim to press on sensitive vaginal walls, making it far more comfortable than the diaphragm. Thus, it can be left in place for several days or longer. The cap stays snugly on the cervix, requiring no extra applications of spermicidal cream or jelly until it is removed. Consequently, it is far less

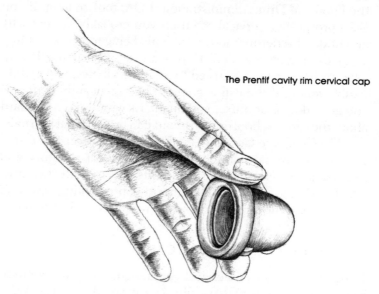

The Prentif cavity rim cervical cap

messy. Some women still prefer to use the cap more or less like a diaphragm, inserting it anywhere from a few minutes to a few hours before they anticipate having intercourse and removing it sometime the next day. Others keep it in for longer periods, and especially like the convenience of being able to keep it in over the weekend.

In spite of its many positive features, early cap users in the United States found that, like all other birth control methods, the cap has its drawbacks as well—similar, for the most part, to those experienced by diaphragm users. Its most immediate and vexing quirk is that not every woman can be fit. The four sizes of the Prentif simply do not accommodate the normal diversity in women's cervical anatomy. There is also considerable variation in fitting criteria. Most practitioners fit about 80 percent of their clients, but some may fit as much as 95 or as little as 50 percent. A few women experience dislodgements which can undermine their confidence in the cap's effectiveness, and some report a buildup of odor inside the cap after leaving it in place for two or three days. Because of variations in individual anatomy, some women's partners can feel the cap in place, but in most cases it is merely an awareness that something is there, rather than discomfort.

One of the unexpected surprises women and their partners have discovered about the cap is its positive impact on sexuality, including a rise in libido and an increase in the frequency of intercourse. With greater freedom from spermicide and the demands of daily insertion and removal, many women appear to *enjoy* using the cap more. "I like the ease I now feel in being able to insert the cap at my leisure, well ahead of any anticipated sexual contact," a New York City actress reports. "I love the freedom to repeat intercourse if I like, or just to go off to sleep without having to deal with any kind of apparatus."

With the reappearance of the cervical cap, some practitioners have noticed a new positive tone in birth control clinics. "Women come into the clinic excited about birth control for a change," reports Deborah Fleming of Womancare in San Diego. "We certainly never observed that with the Pill or the IUD." San Francisco midwife Katy O'Leary reports very enthusiastic responses from cap users: "A full 78.5 percent of the women found the cap extremely satisfactory, and 84 percent preferred it to all other forms of contraception they had used previously." Dr. James Koch, a Brookline, Massachusetts, gynecologist, found that "91 percent . . . were at least moderately, if not completely, satisfied with their caps."

CERVICAL CAP DATA

By now, the Prentif cap has been in use in the United States and parts of Canada as well for nearly a decade. In this time, more than thirty thousand women were fitted with cervical caps under FDA guidelines, and an estimated ten thousand more received caps before the FDA regulation took effect. The cap was always, and continues to be, legal in Canada, but in the United States, it was required to undergo a rigorously controlled scientific study mandated by the FDA and funded by the National Institute of Child Health and Human Development (NICHHD). This $2-million study, comparing the cap to the diaphragm, was conducted in Los Angeles by Dr. Gerald Bernstein, a well-known barrier-method researcher. Completed in March of 1986, the study found the cap to be as effective as the diaphragm. For "typical users," the cap was 82.6 percent effective compared to 83.3 for the diaphragm. For "perfect users," that is, those women who used their caps *for every session of intercourse between menstrual periods with spermicide for one year*, the cap was 94.6 percent effective compared to 96.4 for the diaphragm. The study also revealed that *women overwhelmingly prefer the cervical cap*. One pointed indicator of this preference is the fact that four times as many diaphragm users dropped out of the study as cap users did.

In addition to the NICHHD-funded study, nearly a hundred other cervical cap investigators—including doctors, nurses, nurse practitioners, physicians' assistants, midwives, and an army of trained lay health workers—provided cervical caps on an experimental basis, submitting follow-up data on cap users to the FDA. Many of these practitioners report effectiveness rates in the range of 90 to 96 percent, considerably higher than in the NICHHD-funded study. "No other barrier birth control method has been studied so widely prior to approval," observes Dr. Gary Richwald of the UCLA School of Public Health, who coordinated an in-depth study of more than twenty-five hundred cap users at thirteen study sites in Los Angeles.

Much of the information in this book is based on my own experience as a cervical cap investigator at the Los Angeles Feminist Women's Health Center and Womancap in New York City, and on interviews with nearly one hundred of the practitioners who provided caps on an experimental basis during the FDA study period. The fruits of this survey appear on nearly every page of this guide and some of the results, including effectiveness rates, are summarized on pages 192–196. The willingness of these practitioners to share the results of their work with me, and thus with women and other practitioners, provides a wealth of empirical data on cap use and fitting from a diversity of perspectives. Many of these committed practitioners barely broke even financially after complying with FDA study requirements and received little in the way of professional rewards. Yet, without their foresight and acute awareness of the need for low-risk contraceptive options, the cap would have been completely unavailable during the study period.

THE BIRTH CONTROL CRISIS

The cervical cap burst upon the contraceptive scene at a particularly critical moment: the height of the modern birth control crisis. Not every woman can or will take the Pill and anywhere from 30 to 50 percent of women discontinue its use within the first year because of unwanted effects. And a flood of lawsuits has driven the IUD off of the market. In a larger sense, high-technology contraception, which for the first time in history offered sex without fear of pregnancy, has simply failed to deliver.

A commonly held assumption among family-planning practitioners is that a woman will use an average of three birth control methods during her reproductive life. But this assessment seriously understates the case. A glaring hallmark of the birth control crisis is that more than half of all women who have chosen—or resorted to—surgical sterilization are under the age of thirty, and 20 percent are under twenty-five.* Indeed, by the time they are twenty-five, many women have already tried all available options and still have roughly a quarter of a century of contraceptive use ahead of them. According to one survey, more than 60 percent of women think that *there is no acceptable contraceptive.*† This highly untenable situation is further complicated by the fact that women are increasingly concerned about health risks of chemical contraception, infertility rates associated with IUD use, and the lack of protection from the growing epidemic of sexually transmitted diseases.

In the United States, there are roughly 55 million women of reproductive age, and at any one time about 35 million are in need of birth control. Twelve million women are sterilized or have partners who are. About 10 million women use the Pill, 2.5 million had IUDs at the time its manufacture ceased in the United States, and 3 million women use the diaphragm. Four and a half million women depend on condoms, about 1.5 million women use the contraceptive sponge, and about 1.5 million abortions are performed each year. Thus far, there is no estimate of how cervical cap approval will impact on this market, but it is clear from its recent resurgence that there is strong demand for a new low-risk method.

The women who have sought out the cap prior to FDA approval were a highly self-selected group. Many were current or former diaphragm users who were already comfortable with the concept of inserting a device into the vagina. Others were refugees from the Pill who were no longer willing to tolerate ongoing physical discomfort, or ex–IUD users who suffered medical complications or were concerned about their future fertility. A significant percentage of these women had already been through every available method and were desperately

* Linda E. Atkinson, Richard Lincoln, and Jacqueline Darroch Forrest, "The Next Contraceptive Revolution," *Family Planning Perspectives*, vol. 18, no. 1 (Jan.–Feb. 1986), p. 19.
† Survey by Yankelovich, Shelly and White, 1982. Cited in Atkinson, et al, p. 20.

looking for something they could live with. Although investigational studies included women of various ages and backgrounds, the preponderance were daughters of the baby boom: white, unmarried college graduates in their mid-twenties to late thirties.

"The cervical cap is *the* method for baby boomers," remarks Teri Albright, administrator of the Oakland Feminist Women's Health Center. "They are getting too old to take the Pill, but are still extremely sexually active and want to protect their fertility."

CAP MYTHS

During the years that the cervical cap was under study, most people thought of it as "banned," "illegal," or simply "unavailable" and assumed it would more than likely never be approved. After an initial spate of magazine articles, media excitement about the cap died down, and in the ensuing vacuum a considerable body of mythology developed.

You may have heard one or another of these myths:

The cap is difficult to insert or remove. This myth has been perpetuated mainly by physicians who have never fit caps and by magazine writers who were probably not cap users. The truth is that most new cap users achieve adequate proficiency after just a few minutes of practice. Those who do have difficulty may need several weeks of experience and perhaps a second training session.

The cap can be left in place indefinitely. The fact that women in Victorian times wore the cap during the entire span between the menstrual periods probably accounts for the origin of this widely held notion. Most modern practitioners recommend using the cap for a maximum of three days, but others believe that it can be left in place longer.

Extended cap use might promote cervical cancer. This supposition has no basis in fact, but was fairly widespread in medical circles until recently. "It just doesn't seem like a good idea," doctors often reply when asked to justify their reasoning.

In fact, nearly all of the cervical cap investigators surveyed for this book report *no increase* in cervical irritation, and some have specifically noted protective effects similar to those offered by the diaphragm.

The cap can cause Toxic Shock Syndrome. When the cap first became available in the United States, medical practitioners assumed that there might be some small risk of Toxic Shock Syndrome (TSS) similar to that possible with the use of tampons.* While not nearly enough women have used the cap to allow for even *one* case of TSS, many practitioners feel that the relative risk is exceedingly low, especially if you do not use your cap during menstruation.

There's a "conspiracy" to keep the cap off the market. A political myth about the cap, that perhaps reflects how cynical women and the general public have become about contraception, is that there was somehow an insidious conspiracy between the FDA and drug companies to keep the cap from being approved—to buy time for some U.S. company to come up with a cap of its own. As can be seen in chapter 3, no such conspiracy is evident. The delay in approval can be readily attributed to two major factors: 1) the cap's entanglement in cumbersome bureaucratic regulations that were intended to screen out high-risk devices like heart pacemakers and hip implants and, 2) its manufacturer's reluctance to undertake expensive animal testing to satisfy regulations it views as unnecessary.

HOW TO USE *THE COMPLETE CERVICAL CAP GUIDE*

If the cervical cap is old, low-risk, and simple to use, then why is a book about it necessary? No one, after all, has written a

---

* The risk of getting TSS from tampon use is about one in a million. According to *Contraceptive Technology*, reported cases caused by diaphragm and contraceptive sponge use have not been thoroughly documented.

book solely about the diaphragm, condom, or the contraceptive sponge.

Because the cap has never been used on a large scale in North America, practitioners who do not have any prior experience with the cap and the general public may be skeptical about its safety and effectiveness. The review of the cap's long and venerable history in chapter 2 shows that the cap faded into the background not because it was ineffective, but because it was erroneously believed that the diaphragm was a more efficient method of contraception on a large scale. Chapter 3 relates the details of the cap's rediscovery by feminist clinics and medical practitioners and describes how it and other birth control devices are scrutinized for federal approval.

The information on fitting in chapter 4 is designed to introduce practitioners who are just beginning to fit the cap to the differences in techniques and fitting criteria employed by longtime cap fitters. Most practitioners will probably seek training from an experienced cap fitter, and in this case chapter 4 can serve as a primer to such training. It might also serve as a source of primary material for practitioners who may be in the position of having to learn to fit caps on their own.

Even after the cap is approved by the FDA, not all practitioners will choose to offer it, and you may find it difficult at first to find a qualified fitter in your area. Chapter 5 offers a number of suggestions about how to locate cap clinics and practitioners who provide caps. A list of the investigators who fit caps during the FDA study—and will undoubtedly continue to offer them after approval—appears on page 185.

The cap is not a pill, a fix, or a surgical snip. It is a user-controlled device whose many variations in use may only become apparent after you use it for a while. Because of time limitations, practitioners can provide only a limited amount of information in a clinic setting. Therefore, this book as a whole, especially chapters 4 through 8, can serve as an extra clinic session, offering many details on how to use your cap and advice on how to solve or minimize any problems you may encounter. These chapters contain numerous personal accounts from cap users and reports from practitioners on how women have adapted the cap to their own personal tastes and habits as well as the needs and demands of their partners.

Naturally, women who make use of this guide will be at different stages regarding the cap. If you are contemplating getting a cervical cap, reading through the whole book can offer reassurance that the cap is not some new experimental device, but is a solid, safe, and reliable method of contraception; in addition, it can give you a good idea about what to expect at a cap fitting. If you have just gotten your cap, these chapters might answer questions you forgot to ask your fitter. If you are an experienced cap user, you may find that they contain suggestions for variations in use which may not have occurred to you.

Over half of the teenagers in the United States are sexually active and of those who do use contraception, more than 80 percent take the Pill. Although young women in large numbers have not had an opportunity to try the cervical cap, chapter 9 offers some food for thought for the practitioners who counsel young people on birth control, suggesting that the cap may provide a useful alternative for teenagers who cannot or do not want to take the Pill.

The first thing that women—and practitioners—want to know about any birth control method is how effective it is. Chapter 10 provides information on cap effectiveness from the Bernstein study as well as from nearly one hundred of the cervical cap investigators. Because the efficacy of all birth control methods, especially barriers, varies according to both use and study design, study results can be difficult to interpret. This chapter also includes a brief explanation of the different factors that can influence effectiveness so that the variations in cap rates from the many cap studies might be less confusing.

The decision to try the cervical cap can't be made in a vacuum. It needs to be evaluated in the context of other contraceptive options, your past birth control experiences, your general health, your pattern of sexual activity, your partner's demands, and plans for future children. Chapter 11 offers a survey of all available contraceptive methods to help you compare them with the cap so that your decision is based on the best possible information—both positive and negative—about each of your choices. In addition, the section on fertility awareness can be especially useful in helping you to identify when you can get pregnant, so if you are using the cervical cap or other barrier method, you can decide when not to take risks and how to use any method of birth control far more effectively.

If you are unable to be fit with a Prentif cap, you will surely want to know if other cap models may become available soon. Chapter 12 offers an overview of existing cap designs and current research projects. Tests of several "second-generation" caps are beginning in the foreseeable future, and with luck one or two may be submitted to the FDA for approval within the next five years.

A BARRIER-METHOD RENAISSANCE?

The dramatic reappearance of the cervical cap in the United States represents the first new wrinkle in the contraceptive ball game in thirty years. The Prentif's excellent report card from nearly a hundred practitioners and praise from an overwhelming majority of women dashes the myth that barrier methods are too inconvenient, ineffective, and inelegant to be used on a large scale, and provides concrete directions of inquiry for enterprising cap researchers. Because the cap is low-risk, user-controlled, and has many possible variations in use, it offers real hope to women caught up in the birth control crisis, and with appropriate funding for research and development it has the potential of becoming our most versatile and adaptable contraceptive option.

2 ✳ TRIED AND TRUE:
The 150-Year History of the Cervical Cap

Here begin the medicines to be made whereby a woman might cease to conceive for one, two, or three years: (mix a concoction of certain drugs and honey), moisten lint therewith, and place it at her uterus.*

—*Papyrus Ebers*, Pl. 93, 6–8
(c. 1550 B.C.)

In early Neolithic times, it was thought that women were impregnated by magical, or at least naturalistic, means and little attention was given to the inhibition of this apparently spontaneous process. But once people recognized that depositing sperm in the vagina frequently resulted in pregnancy, perhaps as early as 4000 B.C., the search to control conception had begun. In spite of a profound lack of knowledge about the physiology of conception, primitive cultures devoted considerable energy and creativity to the pursuit of its prevention, relying at first on celibacy, lactation, sexual taboos, and, when these methods failed, crude abortion techniques and infanticide. (All of these methods are practiced today, along with a range of modern drugs and devices.)

Written descriptions of birth control practices date from the time of the Pharaohs, including, among other things, spermicides and a number of commonsensical devices which

---

* Reproduced by permission of Geron-X.

represent the earliest forms of the cervical cap and the contraceptive sponge. The famed Petri medical papyrus, dating from 1850 B.C., describes a pessary or vaginal insert made of dried crocodile dung and *auyt* paste. This malleable, adhesive, porous material might have been pressed around the cervix, serving as a sponge to soak up semen, as well as a homemade, individually fit cervical barrier. The Ebers papyrus, inscribed about 1550 B.C., records the use of medicated lint tampons, which may have killed sperm and served as a physical barrier as well. Jewish women in the first century A.D. heeded a Talmudic admonition to "cohabit with a sponge," while Greek women of the time made use of suppositories and pessaries infused with oily, astringent or acidic substances.

Some of history's most renowned philosophers, from Aristotle and his heirs to the eleventh-century Jewish/Islamic physician Avicenna, have described an astonishing array of contraceptive techniques in discourses upon civilization's eternal quest to inhibit conception. These sundry catalogs include lists of potions, libations, fumigants, magical amulets, and rituals—some of which surely caused a revulsion to sex, in addition to any prophylactic properties they might have had —and enumerate a wealth of naturally occurring spermicidal agents and homemade occlusive devices.

Women of widely disparate cultures have probably used the halves of acidic fruits as natural cervical caps, but the eighteenth-century Italian *bon vivant* Casanova is credited with being the first person to publicly promote the use of the half of a squeezed lemon as a contraceptive method. While it might irritate delicate vaginal mucosa, the highly acidic lemon juice has well-known sperm-killing properties, and the rind might attach itself to the vaginal vault by suction, also serving as a natural barrier.

Prostitutes of nineteenth-century China and Japan covered the cervix with *misugami*, disks of oiled bamboo paper, and Hungarian women fashioned disks of beeswax into disposable do-it-yourself cervical caps. Women of various cultures have also been reported to block the cervical os with balls of opium, which may also have been molded, cap-like, over the cervix. This particular "cervical cap" may have not only prevented conception, but, if its essence were absorbed through the vaginal walls, must have added its own particular gloss to the sexual experience as well.

THE MODERN CERVICAL CAP

It appears that modern cervical caps were developed independently in both Germany and the United States in the nineteenth century, perhaps within a decade or so of each other. The custom-fit German cap was probably not widely used and was supplanted with mass-produced models in the 1880s when higher quality rubber became available. The technology and design of the U.S. model appear to have been lost altogether for almost half a century, due perhaps to aggressive anti-contraceptive laws and puritanical social policy.

The first mention of a modern cervical cap appears in a book entitled *Das weibliche Gebärunvermögen*, by Dr. Friedrich Adolph Wilde, a German anatomy professor, in 1838. Wilde reports that midwives who served rural women appeared to employ some sort of vaginal insert to promote child spacing. In his handbook, Wilde recommends the cervical cap over both the condom and contraceptive sponge, and offers clear directions for its manufacture. "Such persons who are affected with an inability to bear should constantly wear a rubber pessary, which has no opening, which completely covers the os, fits snugly, and which is taken off only during the menses. In order that it may suit every individual case just right, it must be made from a special model made each time by taking a wax impression of the parts by use of a vaginal speculum. This rubber pessary would be less troublesome and uncomfortable than any other kind of cervical cap." *

A homegrown variety of cervical cap may have been invented in the United States in the 1840s or 1860s by Dr. Edward Bliss Foote, an activist physician and popularizer of medical knowledge. A patent for the device was denied, according to Foote, on the grounds that it could be used for

---

* This translation is from Norman N. Himes, *The Medical History of Contraception* (New York: Schocken Books, 1970).

"immoral purposes," and the original model was widely counterfeited. Poor copies, laments the inventor, caused people to become disillusioned with the device and it eventually disappeared from favor.*

Although Foote's invention did not survive, his philosophy of contraception far outstripped medical opinion of his time, and, for that matter, of our own. "It is fair to conclude," he argued, "that the invention of my office for placing the control of reproduction (where it belongs) in the control of the wife, would have been improved, or supplanted by better inventions under proper encouragement . . . from the patent office."

THE CAP IN VICTORIAN ENGLAND

The Victorians were firm believers that the state could and should legislate morality, and vigorously used the legal and medical establishments to suppress the dissemination of birth control information on the grounds that it was obscene. As early as 1830, a few physicians and social activists, working within the incipient population-control movement, began to defy official prohibitions against the dissemination of birth control information. Many of these activists, who called themselves "neo-Malthusians" promoted contraception to limit the poor, lest they, as predicted by economist Thomas

---

* A computer search of several major libraries revealed no copies of Foote's pamphlet *Words in Pearl for the Married* (1876), which reportedly describes his invention as well as other contemporary contraceptive techniques. An oblique reference to the device appears in Foote's 1875 pamphlet, *A Step Backward*, decrying the oppressive censorship of the Comstock laws under which the good doctor himself was prosecuted. "The first reliable means for the use of [the device by] the wife was an invention of my office, having been imperfectly suggested by an associate physician and developed by myself some thirty years ago," Foote wrote. An article by Dr. Hannah M. Stone, the second director of the Margaret Sanger Research Bureau (today the clinical arm of Planned Parenthood in New York City), makes note of an English pamphlet (1892) by a Mr. J. R. Holmes, in which a letter from Foote affirms his invention of a cap in the 1860s, "including a picture and detailed description of the check-pessary." This date is at variance with the mid-1840s date suggested by Foote's 1875 pamphlet, but nonetheless serves to further confirm the existence of a New World cap.

Malthus, increase in number and engulf the rising middle class. Other activists espoused contraception as a health measure as well.

The Wife's Handbook, published in London in 1883 by Dr. Henry Allbutt, contained an advertisement for cervical caps, and an 1887 pamphlet by feminist social activist Annie Besant recommended the India-rubber pessary, or cervical cap, mentioning a certain London pharmacy where the device was readily available.

In Germany, active cervical cap research was under way. In 1908 Dr. K. Kafka, a Viennese gynecologist, designed the "Bimetallkappe," a custom-fit cap, using a plaster cast of the cervix.* In the same year, Kafka published articles on the cap in several German medical journals.

THE MOTHERS OF MODERN BIRTH CONTROL

The heroic, brilliant, and controversial careers of Margaret Sanger and her British counterpart, Marie Stopes, paralleled and sometimes collided with one another. Their courageous and frequently outrageous activities helped to focus attention on the need for contraceptive information, but their unreconstructed eugenic views—espousing contraception especially for the poor and defective—which each held firmly to the end, have prevented them from becoming the authentic heroines that feminists and social activists might have liked. Nonetheless, their single-minded devotion to the cause of women's sexual and reproductive freedom left indelible marks on the history of feminism, the tradition of social activism, and the worldwide population-control movement founded under Sanger's leadership in the late 1920s.

Margaret Sanger is generally assumed to be the first twentieth-century champion of the cervical cap, but the real credit belongs to Emma Goldman. According to historian James Reed, Goldman attended a secret neo-Malthusian conference

* Wolfgang Müller, "Zur Kontrazeption mit Portiokappen." Inaugural-Dissertation zur Erlangung der Doktorwürde in der Zahnheilkunde an der Ludwig Maximilians-Universitat zu München, 1983.

in Paris in 1900 and "returned to the United States with a stock of birth control literature and supplies, determined to make open discussion of contraception a reality."* Goldman subsequently barnstormed the country, advocating the open dissemination of birth control information. At every whistle-stop and public gathering, she distributed a pamphlet entitled "Why the Poor Should Not Have Many Children," which recommended the use of cervical caps, diaphragms, and condoms.

Sanger had her consciousness raised after observing a woman die from an attempted abortion on New York's Lower East Side in 1912, and thereafter dedicated her life to the pursuit of effective birth control. Her inquiries about contraception met only cynicism and silence, if not outright derision from male physicians, so, armed with introductions to the neo-Malthusians supplied by Goldman, she went to England, France, and Holland in search of her Holy Grail—birth control information. She visited the clinic of Dr. Johannes Rutgers at The Hague and discovered "over 15 kinds of devices, including 14 sizes of the *Minsinga* pessary" (the German diaphragm), and found to her amazement that in Holland "contraception was looked upon as no more unusual than we in America look upon the purchase of a tooth brush."†

Sanger's experience at The Hague notwithstanding, the first edition of her famous pamphlet, *Family Limitation*, surreptitiously printed in 1914, contained an illustration of a cervical cap labeled "French pessary—slightly different from the American," and made no mention of the diaphragm. "This is one of the most common preventive articles used in France as well as among the women of the middle and upper class in America," Sanger informed her readers. "In my opinion a well-fit pessary is the surest method of absolutely preventing conception."

* James Reed, *The Birth Control Movement and American Society: From Private Vice to Public Virtue* (Princeton, N.J.: Princeton University Press, 1983). This edition contains a new preface on the relationship between historical scholarship and feminist issues.
† Margaret Sanger, *My Fight for Birth Control* (Elmsford, N.Y.: Maxwell Reprint Co., 1969).

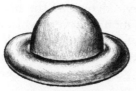

The French pessary recommended by Margaret Sanger in *Family Limitation*, 1916

Mizpah cap

Marie Stopes's Prorace cap or check pessary

Metal cap

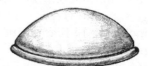

Dutch cap or diaphragm

In 1916, on yet another trip to England, Sanger met Marie Stopes, and introduced her to the cervical cap. "We met again the following week for dinner in her home and inspected and discussed the French pessary which she stated she saw for the first time," Sanger recalls in her autobiography. Stopes, who thought the diaphragm caused "distention of the vaginal muscles," wholeheartedly embraced the cervical cap and designed a special model, which she dubbed the "Prorace" cap or "check pessary." This cap was manufactured by Lambert & Son, predecessor to the present-day Lamberts Ltd.

The Mother's Clinic, founded by Stopes in 1921, never ceased to favor cervical caps. During World War II, when ordinary materials were in short supply, Lamberts made caps for the clinic from a commandeered shipment of rubber intended for the floors of bathrooms in an expensive French hotel. "Those gay caps almost became heirlooms," recalled Dr. Helena Wright, a pioneer British birth control activist, in 1972. "No two caps were alike. . . . marbled patterns of all colors appeared and the rubber lasted so well that even now, here and there, a specimen survives." These colorful objects may have inadvertently been our first designer cervical caps.

Stopes's book, *Birth Control Today*,* contains an eclectic catalog of "good domestic, makeshift methods," even including an ersatz cervical cap made from a child's collapsible rubber ball. The instructions for use include the price of "a penny or twopence each" and read: "Prick it with a thick pin before insertion to let the air out so it doubles back on itself and closes together in the shape of a cap . . . such a collapsible ball should be placed as nearly like a cap as possible."

It is not clear precisely when Sanger changed her allegiance from the cervical cap to the diaphragm. Certainly her visit to Holland, where the diaphragm was universally preferred, must have been influential. For a time, she and some friends imported illegal diaphragms through Canada in cartons marked "Three-in-One-Oil," a product manufactured by Noah Slee, Sanger's wealthy second husband. But smuggling proved too arduous a task in the long run, and imported spermicides were of uneven quality. At Sanger's behest, Slee funded the establishment of the Holland Rantos Company in 1925, which produced the first domestically manufactured diaphragms and spermicide.

In spite of a preference for the diaphragm by Sanger and her friends in the neo-Malthusian League, Dr. Robert Latou Dickinson, a New York gynecologist, "visited main surgical supply houses in German-speaking countries in 1926, and found that sales of caps of metal and celluloid had displaced sales of rubber diaphragms four to one." Dr. Hans Lehfeldt confirms that during the 1920s and 1930s, more than fifty models of the cervical cap were available in Europe, and they were preferred by women and physicians alike. During the

* Marie Carmichael Stopes, *Birth Control Today* (London: The Hogarth Press, 1957).

European heyday of the cervical cap, a variety of metal caps, and an ill-fated ivory model, were also produced by Russian researchers.

In 1931, Dr. Walter Pust, a gynecologist from Wittenberg, Germany, confirmed the widespread use of the cervical cap in Germany. "About eight years ago, I began prescribing celluloid caps for the treatment of cervical troubles, erosions and gonorrhea. When I inquired into the question, about five or six years later, I found that these caps were being used as the most usual method of contraception. In addition to the specially authorized factory, four others had been set up which produced copies of the authorized cap so that, judging by the figures I was able to obtain, it appeared that from 500,000 to 600,000 caps had been sold. This led me to believe that the model must be good otherwise it would not have been copied."*

U.S. MODELS

Although the cervical cap never caught fire in the United States, it apparently survived in disparate quarters. Dr. Rachelle S. Yarros, a gynecologist on the staff at Chicago's Hull House, published a brief report in 1927 asserting that she provided "nothing but a French Pessary" in her practice for nearly thirty years.† In the 1930s, Dr. Bessie L. Moses, a Baltimore gynecologist, described successful use of a cervical cap with "a very thin rubber dome and a flange or flat rim which is attached to the dome at a very slight angle," manufactured by Durex Products. Another cap—the Cervicap—of silver (six sizes), chrome (twelve sizes), firm amber plastic (nine sizes), and clear softer plastic or rubber (nine sizes) was made by the Surgical Instrument Research Laboratory in New York City. According to a pamphlet produced by the manufacturer, the Cervicaps were exhibited at the National Conference on Birth Control in Washington in 1934, and were

* Margaret Sanger and Hannah M. Stone, *The Practice of Contraception* (Baltimore: The Williams and Wilkins Co., 1931), p. 24.
† Sanger and Stone, p. 17.

being provided on a limited basis by the Margaret Sanger Research Bureau in New York City.

In addition to the elaborate array of Cervicaps, two domestic manufacturers, Ortho Pharmaceuticals and Milex-Western, sold hard plastic caps beginning in the 1940s. Later, both companies designated their products primarily as devices useful for holding sperm next to the cervix in artificial insemination and put little effort into their marketing as birth control devices.

This scattered activity notwithstanding, from the mid-1930s on, the term "cervical cap" all but disappeared from the contraceptive lexicon in the United States. Throughout the 1940s and 1950s couples depended heavily upon condoms and withdrawal or, if they sought the advice of a physician, the diaphragm.

More than any other single individual, Dr. Hans Lehfeldt has kept faith with the cervical cap. Lehfeldt, whose career as a gynecologist began in Berlin in 1923, worked closely with the stalwarts of the original birth control movement, including Sanger and Stopes, Havlock Ellis, and Drs. Ernest Grafenberg, Christopher Tietze, and Robert Latou Dickinson. When he fled Germany before the Nazi takeover, Lehfeldt set up practice in New York City and, in 1958, founded the first birth control clinic in a municipal hospital in the United States at New York City's Bellevue Hospital. Lehfeldt used domestic caps made by Ortho and Milex-Western and went to Europe several times each year, returning with a suitcase full of cervical caps made in Germany or Denmark. When the Pill came on the market and Ortho announced it would no longer produce its plastic cap, Lehfeldt "bought up the company's entire supply so that I could continue to provide them in the clinic." Although he retired from the clinic in 1972, Lehfeldt continued to provide European hard plastic caps in his practice until the FDA forbade their importation in 1980. During that time, he may have been the only physician in the United States to dispense the orphan devices.

WHAT REALLY HAPPENED TO
THE CERVICAL CAP?

In 1988 the modern cervical cap in its many guises will be 150 years old. As we look back, its history is as surprising in its breadth and depth as is its brush with extinction. Now that the cap has made a dramatic reappearance in North America, everyone is wondering just what happened to this handy little device.

The diaphragm came into its own in Holland, where contraception was considered a routine health measure. Although the cap was widely used in both Germany and France, it came of age in Victorian England, where it was considered inappropriate for women to deal with genital matters. Individual women bought caps in apothecary shops or ordered them by mail, but women of means often had them inserted by their physicians after their menstrual periods and removed again just before the onset of bleeding. This mode of provision established the cap's reputation as a "physician-controlled" device and apparently accompanied the British activists who attended the early international birth control conferences held in Europe. On the other hand, the Dutch view of the diaphragm as a device easily handled by women themselves had many proponents at these early conferences.

Drs. Grafenberg and Dickinson, two committed birth control activists, confirm the philosophical drift toward the diaphragm in an article promoting cap use in the United States in 1944. "All protection against unwise pregnancy has as a primary desirability that the means be placed in the hands of the woman herself. It is largely on this account that the rubber vaginal diaphragm has won its front rank among physicians." Nonetheless, the cap continued to be a popular method of birth control in England and held its own in the United States well into the 1930s, where it was provided, along with the diaphragm, at the Margaret Sanger Research Bureau.*

---

* Dr. Hannah Stone, the bureau's longtime director, indicated a slight preference for the diaphragm in *The Practice of Contraception*, but noted, "We believe both [the cap and the diaphragm] have their individual indica-

Focus on the diaphragm was not based upon scientific data, but upon experiential information that was highly colored by social values and the developing philosophy of population controllers whose sights were set on a single goal: contraception on a massive scale. However well-intentioned their motives, Sanger and her cohorts in the population-control movement saw the diaphragm as a more direct route to contraception and they promoted it with vigor, to the neglect of an equally useful and more convenient method, the cervical cap. Sanger never repudiated the cervical cap, however, and continued to think of it as a useful option for individual women.

But by the mid-1970s, what was already all too apparent to women became clear to feminists, consumer advocates, and a few progressive medical practitioners—that high-tech birth control was failing to live up to its promise and that a crisis was indeed at hand. Pill use began to decline due to adverse publicity about potential hazards, the Dalkon Shield scandal broke, and no new methods appeared forthcoming. So advocates of an alternative to existing methods looked into the past, scratched the surface, and found, without having to look very far, the cervical cap. They then set about debunking the Victorian myth, which still lurks in the corner of gynecologists' offices like the faint smell of disinfectant, that the cap is more difficult for women to use.

---

tions." In the *Journal of Contraception* in 1937 she stated that "it takes hardly any more time to instruct a woman how to insert a cervical cap as to teach her the use of a diaphragm." Cited in Deborah Boehm, "The Cervical Cap: Effectiveness as a Contraceptive," *Journal of Nurse-Midwifery* 28, no. 1 (Jan.–Feb. 1983), pp. 3–6.

3 ✳ THE CERVICAL CAP RENAISSANCE:
Perhaps Our Foremothers Knew Best

> The cervical cap is guerrilla contraception; it is a neat, elegant and economic solution to the contraception problem and it can be made to work again.
>
> —Germaine Greer
> *Sex and Destiny*

Interest in the cervical cap seems to have sprung up simultaneously and spontaneously in widely disparate areas of both the United States and Canada, almost as if some kind of critical mass had been reached. As the realities of the birth control crisis began to sink in, health activists and concerned practitioners were on the lookout for developments in contraception, although they knew that the prospects for new, low-risk options were not hopeful.

In 1977, Barbara Seaman included a chapter on the cervical cap in *Women and the Crisis in Sex Hormones*, a book that became the definitive work on the modern birth control crisis. In researching alternatives to the Pill, she had traveled to England and interviewed an aristocratic mother of four, identified in the book as "Lady R," who generously shared the details of her lifelong use of the cervical cap. Seaman also included the experience of a New York friend who had, for many years, used a silver European pessary. Looking to the future, the book proposed that "clinics and women's health centers will start ordering caps from England, and that American firms will soon resume manufacture." Later, when the modest cervical cap renaissance that she proposed came to pass, the information in *Women and the Crisis in Sex Hormones* became an invaluable reference for practitioners and women who were interested in trying the cap. Seaman's authoritative advocacy of the cap also helped influence its acceptance as a potentially important birth control option.

THE CERVICAL CAP PIONEERS

At roughly the same time that the Seamans' book appeared, Nurse Practitioner Irene Snair came across brief mention of the cervical cap in a textbook used in a course on human sexuality she took in the fall of 1976.* Snair, who was assistant director of the Student Health Service at New England College in Henniker, New Hampshire, thought the cap might have possibilities. She wrote to Lamberts asking for information and talked to Dr. John Bently, a co-worker at the Student Health Service who had fit caps in England. He assured her that they were not difficult to fit, so she decided to order some and try them out. Her experiment was a success and in September of 1977 Snair began providing caps at the Student Health Service and in her private practice. Snair was the first of the new wave of cap providers in the United States and became a pivotal figure in the revival of this almost-forgotten contraceptive device.

One of the first women Snair fit was Sarah Berndt, a nursing student who worked part-time at the New Hampshire Feminist Health Center in Concord. Berndt introduced the cap to the staff at the health center, and her advocacy was a critical link in its early acceptance and promotion by the women's health movement, which was ultimately responsible for the cap's wide availability during the FDA study period.

On another front, sometime early in 1977, Dr. James Koch, a Brookline, Massachusetts, gynecologist, had a conversation with Dr. Philip Stubblefield of the Harvard School of Public Health about the dearth of viable barrier methods of contraception. Stubblefield mentioned the cervical cap and suggested that it might be interesting to try it out. Koch ordered some Prentifs from Lamberts and began fitting them in December of 1977. He quickly became convinced that the

* Herant A. Katchadourian and Donald T. Lunde, *Fundamentals of Human Sexuality*, 2d ed. (New York: Henry Holt & Co., 1972).

cervical cap was an important, if not vital, concept and began designing new, improved versions in his head. In 1982, Koch published the first medical study on the cap since 1953, hired a biomedical engineer, and set up shop in a back room of his office, hoping to turn his designs into reality.

In July of 1978, the Boston Women's Health Book Collective, the authors of Our Bodies, Ourselves (OBOS), included an article on the cap in a periodic packet of health information circulated to about four hundred women's health activists. This article, based on research done by the collective staff and written by Judith Brillman, offered some of the most detailed information available on the cap at the time and was widely photocopied and passed around among new cap providers.

THE CERVICAL CAP BRIGADE

On May 31, 1978, the New Hampshire Feminist Health Center, located in Concord, held a regional workshop on the cervical cap which included doctors, family-planning practitioners, and women's health organizations from New Hampshire, Massachusetts, and Vermont. The group also conducted workshops in schools, clinics, and conferences and soon became known as the "Cervical Cap Brigade."

"We know the perfect method doesn't exist, but we're talking about options," staff member Betty Mitchell observed. "And it's exciting to be able to offer women more of a choice." * In July of 1978, the clinic began offering caps in its birth control clinic.

When Nurse Practitioner Renee Potik, who worked at the Westside Women's Clinic in Santa Monica, California, read about the cap in the OBOS packet, she picked up the phone and called Irene Snair to learn more and was so intrigued that she immediately flew to New Hampshire for training. Soon Potik began to spread the word to other progressive health care providers in Los Angeles, including lay health workers from the Los Angeles Feminist Women's Health Center. This

* Alice Downey, "Cervical Cap Workshop Held," Womanwise, Summer 1978.

clinic is part of a federation that at one time included seven clinics which ultimately fit more than twenty thousand caps —half of all of the caps dispensed in the United States before FDA approval.

Several staff members from the New Hampshire clinic took caps with them to the annual meeting of the National Abortion Federation in San Francisco on September 24 and 25, 1978. They held a cervical cap workshop attended by physicians, nurse practitioners and representatives of a number of feminist clinics. Many of the workshop's participants returned home and ordered caps from Lamberts, and one after another added this new option to their meager selection of birth control resources. With this event the cervical cap renaissance had truly begun.

"By January, 1979, there were approximately 100 cap providers nationwide and by 1980, this figure had doubled," reports *Womanwise*, the quarterly newsletter of the New Hampshire Feminist Health Center. The publication estimates that in the year and a half since Irene Snair ordered the first caps from England, between ten and fifteen thousand women had sought out practitioners who provided cervical caps.

Soon, the National Women's Health Network, a women's health advocacy organization based in Washington, D.C., devoted space in its newsletter to information on the cervical cap and assembled a nationwide listing of cervical cap providers in answer to queries about availability.

CONTRACAP

Even before these first stirrings of the cervical cap revival which focused on the use of existing models, a chance conversation between dentist Robert Geopp and gynecologist Uwe Freese, colleagues at the University of Chicago School of Medicine, resulted in the idea for a custom-fit cervical cap. The two discussed a patient of Freese's—a forty-year-old woman whose birth control options had just run out: she could no longer use the Pill and found other existing methods unsuitable. Geopp, who is of European origin, suggested the cervical cap, but Freese knew little about them and thought that they had a tendency to fall out. Geopp suggested making custom-fit caps in the way that dentists commonly make custom-fit dental appliances. The two soon formed a company and began experimenting with dental materials, casting techniques, and space-age plastics. The collaboration eventually resulted in the development of the Contracap, an extended-wear cap with a one-way tunnel which allows secretions to seep out. (See page 178 for a description of this cap, which is still in development.)

These disparate threads of interest in the cervical cap arose independently of each other in a period of three short years in response to the growing pressure of the birth control crisis. In spite of modest intentions, the work of early cap providers helped to revive the ebbing belief in barrier methods and unwittingly stimulated interest in further cervical cap research.

THE VIMULE CONTROVERSY

The Vimule cap, also manufactured by Lamberts Ltd., was originally included in the Bernstein study and offered as an alternative by more than one third of the cervical cap investigators. But early on, Linda Kilzer, a nurse working on the Bernstein project, discovered a small cut in the vagina of one of the women who was using a Vimule. All of the eleven study participants who were using this cap were then examined and four—or about 35 percent—had small nicks or cuts in their vaginas which appeared to have been made by the rough edge of the cap.

At the FDA's request, all cap providers asked Vimule users to return for examinations. Of those who returned, about 10 to 15 percent had similar occurrences, a much smaller percentage than originally reported by Bernstein. On the basis of these findings, the FDA issued an order forbidding the further use of the Vimule cap.

Citing the need for further research on the Vimule, the Chelsea Women's Health Team and the Federation of Feminist Women's Health Centers requested a hearing before the FDA to protest the summary discontinuation of the Vimule study. They suggested that instead of dropping this cap from study *before* the risks were thoroughly known and documented, its length of use be modified to twenty-four hours in accordance with the manufacturer's instructions (all women in the Bernstein study had worn the cap for forty-eight hours or more) and more intensive follow-up be done for all Vimule users.

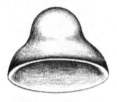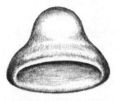

Vimule cap with sharp edge (left)
and suggested modification with blunt edge (right)

The FDA denied the petition and ultimately prohibited further provision of the cap. Some critics of the FDA's action suggested that cuts and tissue buildup caused by the Vimule are similar to the callus-like formations that occur in the mouths of people who wear braces and other dental appliances—that in fact they are expected and that the FDA was overreacting to a hypothetical problem.

Dr. George Denniston, a Seattle gynecologist who published one of the earliest medical studies on the Prentif in 1982, voiced his opposition, saying, "I think it is outrageous that the FDA discontinued research on the Vimule based on the flimsy evidence they had from Bernstein's study." Dr. Koch designed a Vimule with a smooth edge, and turned out some prototypes, but it was never studied.

Barbara Seaman was a strong opponent of further use of the Vimule, fearing that adverse publicity about this cap might reflect on the Prentif's chances to be approved.

A number of other cap investigators asked Lamberts if it would modify the Vimule, but to no avail. P. P. W. Watkins, former administrator of Lamberts,* responded that there had

---

* Lamberts was sold in early 1979.

been no reports of problems with this cap in all of the years that it had been on the worldwide market and that the company had no intention of undertaking the expensive process of recasting the mold. He pointed out that no women in the Bernstein study had used the cap according to the directions on the package insert, which specify that the cap be worn, like the diaphragm, for twenty-four hours.

Before the Vimule controversy arose, many cap providers liked the cap and felt it was a solid alternative for some of the women who could not be fit with a Prentif. Even after the discovery that the rough edge caused some minor injuries, some still felt that it was a very worthwhile option that needed slight modification, either in its design or in its mode of use. (For more information on the Vimule cap, see page 174.)

THE DEVICE AMENDMENTS

The entry of the cervical cap into the contraceptive marketplace is unique. No powerful drug company funded its development and shepherded it through the federal review process, and no well-oiled lobbying agency championed its cause. The truth is that the cervical cap very nearly failed to get approved because most of its U.S. advocates did not understand the finer points of the approval process and its English manufacturer balked at what it considered the unnecessary demands of FDA regulations. A review of the cap's journey through the channels of federal review offers an instructive case study in how drugs and devices in general are approved—or killed— and sheds some light on the current crisis and the future of contraception in the United States.

In the wake of the Dalkon Shield scandal, Congress enacted the Medical Device Amendments of the Federal Food, Drug and Cosmetic Act, mandating the Center for Devices and Radiological Health to "assure the safety, effectiveness and proper labeling of medical devices."* The amendments

* *Everything You Always Wanted to Know about the Medical Device Amendments . . . and Weren't Afraid to Ask*, U.S. Department of Health and Human Services, Pamphlet HHS no. (FDA) 84-4173, 2d ed.

provide three classifications for new devices intended for human use. Class I includes those devices for which sufficient information exists "to assure safety and effectiveness." Class II devices are those for which clarification is needed, but for which "existing information is sufficient to establish a *performance standard*" assuring safety and effectiveness. Class III regulates devices "for which insufficient information exists to assure . . . safety and effectiveness." Generally, Class III devices are those represented as *"life sustaining or life supporting, those implanted in the body, or those presenting potential unreasonable risk of illness or injury"* (emphasis added).

At the time that the Device Amendments were enacted, devices that were already "on the market," such as the diaphragm and the condom, were "grandparented in" (approved provisionally) and later classified and granted final approval.

Because of the cap's extended history and lack of reported problems, its early supporters assumed that it would be quickly approved, but they were wrong. Just about a year after the amendments were enacted, at roughly the same time Irene Snair and James Koch started providing caps, the cap's fate was sealed by the FDA Advisory Committee which was charged with recommending classification and approval or disapproval for devices already "on the market." As a routine matter, the committee, meeting on November 20, 1977, considered the classification of the only cervical cap it could find, the Milex-Western hard plastic cervical cap.

In the years since cap use in the United States had waned, Milex-Western continued to manufacture a plastic cap, but promoted its use only for menstrual collection and as an aid to artificial insemination. For these two purposes, the committee designated cervical caps *as they were currently used in the United States* as Class II, but decided that for any "new intended uses," i.e., contraception, the Milex cap and any other cervical cap should be placed into Class III. The "unreasonable risk" the cap posed was, according to this panel of experts, *pregnancy*. The Milex company, or the manufacturer of any new cap, would therefore have to submit a Premarket Approval (PMA) application before their product could be approved and marketed.

On November 28, 1977, the FDA sent a letter to Lamberts Ltd. asking if its caps were being marketed in the United States. If Lamberts had replied in the affirmative, which it did not, the cap would have been eligible to be "grandparented in" as the diaphragm and condom were. It would probably have been subjected to less stringent standards and placed in the Class II category. In a reply dated December 7, 1977, Lamberts reported that its caps were not on the market in the United States as of May 31, 1976, the date on which the Device Amendments were enacted. The upshot of the negative reply from Lamberts was that the cap was required to go through the arduous Premarket Approval process designed to evaluate such high-risk devices as IUDs, heart pacemakers, and hip implants.

The FDA was blissfully unaware of the Prentif's reappearance upon the scene until Barbara Seaman testified before the Senate Health Subcommittee chaired by Senator Kennedy in August 1979. The topic of the hearing was Depo-Provera, but Seaman talked about the cap as well, urging federal authorities to fund cervical cap research. Her statements at the hearing made the papers, the FDA became apprised of a "new intended use" of the cervical cap, and the bureaucratic wheels began to turn.

In a survey of cervical cap providers conducted by Dana Gallagher of the Vermont Women's Health Center, 80 percent of the respondents were "overwhelmingly in disagreement with the FDA's classification of cervical caps as a Class III device." * Almost without exception, the cervical cap investigators felt that the cap was as safe as the diaphragm and probably at least as effective. There were no indications of any unhealthy effects, and compared to approved methods such as the Pill and IUDs, the cap's potential for causing illness or injury appeared minimal.

In the winter of 1980, cap providers became aware of the cap's new legal status, not by reading the *Federal Register*,

---

* Dana Gallagher, "The Cervical Cap: Issues in the Food and Drug Administration's Regulatory Approval System," Master's Thesis, UCLA School of Public Health, 1986.

where such actions are formally announced, but through the seizure of cap shipments by U.S. Customs officials. "This was the first clue we had that the FDA intended to regulate the cap," Teri Albright of the Oakland Feminist Women's Health Center recalls. "It was a big shock."

At a meeting called by the Department of Health, Education and Welfare—predecessor of the Department of Health and Human Services—to discuss funding of a cervical cap study, Koch and Lehfeldt led the opposition to the proposed Class III designation, but failed to make any headway. As a result of the meeting, however, the FDA requested the National Institute of Child Health and Human Development to fund a study comparing the cap to the diaphragm. The contract was won by Dr. Gerald Bernstein and the study, projected to take four years, was begun on July 1, 1981. It soon became clear that the FDA was immovable on the issue of the cap's classification. Resigned to the fact, cap advocates dug in for the long haul, assuming that the cap could be approved on the strength of positive results from the Bernstein study. But again, they were wrong.*

Because of the Class III designation, Lamberts was required to submit a Premarket Approval application before the cap could be approved for general distribution in the United States. The fly in the ointment, so to speak, was that the PMA requires the submission of clinical, laboratory, *and animal data*, and no animal studies had ever been done on the sixty-year-old Prentif. The quibble turned out to be not effectiveness, or even the material—latex rubber—from which the caps are made, but the color additives and stabilizers used in curing the rubber.

Lamberts submitted specifications on the manufacture of its caps to the FDA, but because such information is considered "proprietary"—i.e., "owned" by the company—the agency could not make use of it in the review process. So, even though the FDA had information on additives to the cap

---

* A thorough chronicle of this phase of the cap's sojourn through governmental channels by Sandra Malasky and Susan Jordan appeared in *Womanwise*, Spring 1981.

material *and* four years of data on the cap's use by women—from the Bernstein study and nearly one hundred other cap investigators as well—it insisted on the letter of the law regarding animal studies. As the Bernstein study grew to a close, reporting no adverse changes in cervical or vaginal health caused by the cap, the FDA dropped the bomb. *It would not accept a PMA from Lamberts without the inclusion of animal data.*

"My understanding is that the whole rationale for animal tests is to set up guidelines for human studies, and not the other way around," says Erica Gollub, who fit cervical caps as a member of the Chelsea Women's Health Team in New York City for six years. "What can they possibly learn from three-month studies that we don't already know from five years of human studies?"

Dr. Lillian Yin, director of the FDA's Center for Devices and Radiological Health, explains the official rationale behind the demand for animal studies. "We know what is going to happen in four or five years, but we don't know what might occur after a 20-year-old woman uses the cap for fifteen years. Maybe there is something in the rubber that could cause a problem. With intensified exposure in rats and mice, we can extrapolate if reactions occur."

Lamberts initially refused to do the studies, citing the lack of any reported problems in more than sixty years of Prentif use and the expense of conducting such studies—in excess of $50,000. "It does seem strange that the FDA wants animal data for something that has been in use for more than sixty years and is approved by the Family Planning Association of Great Britain and the International Planned Parenthood Federation (IPPF), says P. P. W. Watkins.* For a while, because of Lamberts' apparent intransigence, prospects for cap approval appeared bleak indeed.

---

* Planned Parenthood Federation of America, which we all know as "Planned Parenthood," is one of the members of the International Planned Parenthood Federation, but the two are distinct organizations.

FEMINISTS TO THE RESCUE

When it became apparent that the FDA was going to hold the low-risk cervical cap to the same standards that had been established for intrauterine and other high-risk devices, and that its manufacturer refused to go along with what it saw as a useless and expensive exercise, the cap's supporters became concerned. A number of proponents contacted Lamberts in person as well as by phone and mail, urging that the company seek to comply with the FDA requirements and submit the PMA. But Lamberts stood firm. The cap is only a minor product of this small British firm, and more than $50,000 required to execute the animal studies seemed out of line.

Then, in the spring of 1985, public opinion researcher Susan Jordan, aided by Sybil Shainwald (who, as well as Jordan, has done outstanding health advocacy work) and Judy Norsegian of the Boston Women's Health Book Collective, decided to try to break the impasse. Jordan sought to broker an agreement between Lamberts and the FDA over the animal studies. After meeting with Dr. Yin at the FDA and conducting some lengthy negotiations with Lamberts, they succeeded. The FDA agreed to require minimal three-month toxicity studies instead of the two year carcinogenicity studies which it could have demanded, and Lamberts agreed to hire an outside company to conduct the studies. Jordan then began an intensive search for a consultant to locate a suitable company to do the animal studies and expedite the filing of the PMA for Lamberts. She found Environ Corporation, a small Washington, D.C., medical consulting firm which specializes in filing PMA applications. The firm located a company to perform the requisite animal studies and designed protocols for the tests according to FDA specifications.

Many health activists, including Jordan, applaud the thorough review process the cap was forced to undergo and feel that had an exception been made for the cervical cap, other more risky devices might be able to slip through. Others point out that the comparative study with the diaphragm took far too long and was, in fact, unnecessary, and feel that the cap was held up to standards that had been established to screen out high-risk devices.

In a paper written for the *Health/PAC Bulletin*, Erica Gollub suggests that the FDA decided to "make an example of the cap. . . . Both to protect its own reputation and to suggest better protection of the American consumer, the FDA is demonstrating its ability to hold up a product indefinitely at the pre-approval level, through the meticulous application of rules that the FDA typically finds burdensome and rarely applies to the letter."* Some critics have taken a more cynical view, suggesting that officials at the FDA are still smarting from criticism by feminists and consumer advocates for failing to act swiftly when the dangers of the Dalkon Shield became known and are determined not to be caught appearing lax again regarding contraception—an issue which has a vocal and influential advocacy group.

Certainly the Device Amendments provide crucial safeguards in protecting people from medical devices and women from unnecessarily risky contraceptives. But the strict interpretation of their provisions may be preventing much-needed low-risk contraceptives from reaching the marketplace, and may also act to inhibit future research.

CHRONOLOGY OF THE CERVICAL CAP RENAISSANCE

1975	Drs. Robert Geopp and Uwe Freese form partnership to develop Contracap.
1977	Publication of *Women and the Crisis in Sex Hormones.*
Sept. 1977	Irene Snair fits caps at New England College.
Nov. 1977	FDA Advisory Committee designates caps as a Class III device for *contraceptive use.*
Nov. 20, 1977	Letter from FDA to Lamberts Ltd. asking if its cervical caps were "on the market" as of May 31, 1976.
Dec. 1977	James Koch fits caps in Brookline, Massachusetts.

* Erica Gollub, "The Cervical Cap: Test Case for U.S. Regulatory Politics," *Health/PAC Bulletin* 16 (6), Aug. 1986.

Dec. 7, 1977	Lamberts replies to FDA saying that its cap was "not on the market" in the United States as of May 31, 1976.
July 1978	New Hampshire Feminist Health Center begins fitting cervical caps in Concord.
Aug. 1, 1978	Barbara Seaman testifies before Kennedy committee about the cervical cap.
Sept. 24–26, 1978	New Hampshire Feminist Health Center holds workshop on cervical caps at the National Abortion Federation annual meeting in San Francisco.
Nov. 1979	The National Institutes of Health (NIH) calls a meeting to evaluate the need for a federally funded study of the cap.
Jan. 19, 1980	FDA places announcement in the *Federal Register*, making importation of caps illegal except under an Investigational Device Exemption. U.S. Customs begins seizing cap shipments.
July 1, 1981	Bernstein study begins.
March 1982	FDA notifies IDE holders of Bernstein findings regarding Vimule cap.
May 1983	Cervical cap symposiums in Atlanta, Los Angeles, and Seattle sponsored by the Federation of Feminist Women's Health Centers.
Feb. 14, 1984	FDA orders all IDE holders to cease providing Vimule.
Sept. 13–14, 1984	Feminist Women's Health Centers and Chelsea Women's Health Team appeal discontinuation of Vimule at FDA hearings.
Oct. 1984	Appeal of Vimule ruling denied.
Mar. 31, 1985	Bernstein study completed.
June 1986	Results of Bernstein study submitted to NICHHD.
Sept. 1986	Animal studies on Prentif begin.
Dec. 1986	Animal studies on Prentif completed.

4 ✷ THE CERVICAL CAP FITTING:
A Guide for Users and Practitioners

Until Dr. James Koch's comprehensive two-part article appeared in *Contraception* in February 1982, the only published information on cap fitting appeared in *Control of Conception*, a textbook on birth control by Dr. Robert Latou Dickinson published in 1938.* As the cap renaissance spread across the United States, early pioneers, often working in isolation, learned to fit caps by trial and error, practicing on themselves, friends, colleagues, and clients. As they became more confident of their abilities, they began training others, passing on not only fitting skills, but a philosophy of cap provision that differs significantly from the standard medical model.

The cap's first practitioners quickly realized that there is much more to a cap fitting than to the standard five-minute diaphragm visit. They discovered that there are considerably more variables in a cap's fit and that judgments are far more subjective than those required in fitting a diaphragm. The first cap practitioners saw that in order to be effective, fitting a cap and training a woman in its use has to be a completely cooperative effort between client and practitioner. As they worked with women to evaluate fit and to teach insertion and removal skills, many abandoned the standard props of gynecology—stirrups and drape—and invited their clients' active participation in their own fittings.

* Robert Latou Dickinson, *Control of Conception* (Baltimore: The Williams and Wilkins Co., 1938).

The first wave of cap providers also discovered, to no one's surprise, that it does not require a medical degree to fit caps expertly. After basic training and some fitting experience, patience and the quality of client education are the key elements in the competent provision of the cervical cap. It also became apparent very early that fitting a cap properly is necessary, but not sufficient. A woman must also be given confidence that the cap will protect her from pregnancy. In this regard, it is interesting to note that physicians have not necessarily produced higher effectiveness rates than nurse practitioners or clinics staffed by trained lay health workers.

INFORMATIONAL COUNSELING

As interest in the cervical cap spread, practitioners found themselves in the position of having to do a great deal of public education about the device. Many found that telephone counseling or the prior provision of written materials saved an enormous amount of time and energy. Offering basic information ahead of time also helped women to self-select themselves as good candidates for cap use to some extent and gave them a more realistic idea about what to expect from a cap visit.

Because of the increased demand on staff time that providing cervical caps takes, some practitioners have made very effective use of pre-appointment group educational sessions which are separate from the cap fittings. The Washington Women's Self-Help holds monthly "cervical cap teach-ins," which last up to two hours and are often attended by twenty to thirty women. Usually, one or more of the staff members is a cap user herself and contributes her own experiences to the discussion.

Canadian physician Betty Schofield, who reported on a cap study she conducted at the Foothills Hospital in Calgary, Alberta, in 1982, also had excellent results with the monthly group format. At the end of each session, a nurse took a health history, Pap smear, and vaginal culture from women who wanted to make an appointment. Each woman was also given an opportunity to see her cervix. "This . . . was a new and rewarding experience for most women and provided an excellent opportunity to show them where the cap should be placed," Dr. Schofield says. "If the woman was unfamiliar with locating her own cervix, she was encouraged to practice this before her fitting appointment."

THE FITTING SESSION

As caps have come to be fit in the United States, several slight variations in fitting practices have emerged. Some practitioners do the fitting themselves, then supervise each woman as she practices insertion and removal. Others combine the fitting and practice session, allowing a woman to insert each cap herself, and then remove it after the fit has been checked. Many medically trained practitioners still do all counseling, fitting, and training by themselves, but others spread the work among several staff members. Dr. Lehfeldt, for example, fits the caps himself, then while each woman practices insertion and removal, his judgment is checked by two trained assistants.

In some feminist clinics, two trained lay health workers share all of the responsibilities for group sessions and both check each cap, seeking to arrive at a consensus regarding fit. A peek into the exam room of a group fitting session reveals a rather ungynecological scene. The room is typically furnished with couches, and a few chairs, and perhaps strewn with pillows. Five or six women in varying stages of undress can be observed, reclining, squatting, kneeling, or standing, performing the ritual contortions of new cap initiates.

"A few women are leery of group fittings, but after the experience, many appreciate the warmth and support they get from the other women," says Dido Hasper, a director of the Chico, California, Feminist Women's Health Center. "With the amount of information we generally give, it's just not feasible to do it any other way."

Whether you have an individual or a group fitting, your cap visit may be quite different—even more interesting and informative—than the traditional diaphragm fitting. It may be more like a visit to the optometrist. A New York editor who uses the cervical cap notes some striking similarities between her cap visit and a fitting for contact lenses:

> The doctor measured my eye and he inserted the lense for the first time. Then I had to wait one-half hour for my eyes to adjust to the lense. After that, I was sent to an assistant in a back room who helped me learn to insert and remove them and taught me how to clean them with sterile solution. She told me to come back if I had any problems and mentioned that some people come back several times before they are completely comfortable with their lenses. I was there for about an hour.
>
> In contrast, my cap fitting was less complicated. My health worker talked about the cap for a few minutes and explained how to identify fertile mucus. She showed me how to use a speculum and I looked at my cervix. Then she suggested that I try on a size 28 cap. It fit perfectly, but I tried on the size 25 and 31 for comparison. The whole visit took about 45 minutes and I learned more than I ever have from any doctor's visit.

As with fitting contact lenses, diaphragms, or any other kind of device, it is important to take as much time as is necessary to make sure that each woman is comfortable with its use and feels free to return for further help if she experiences problems.

THE ESSENTIALS OF CAP FITTING

While fitting caps and diaphragms differs considerably in certain respects, the prelude to the actual fitting is quite similar to what would be done at a typical diaphragm visit:

- Helping a woman locate her cervix visually and manually
- Taking a Pap smear, gonorrhea culture, and vaginal smears to check for asymptomatic infections or to identify visible symptoms
- Performing a visual exam of the vagina and cervix to ascertain its approximate size and angle and to check for irri-

tation, discoloration, herpes sores, and Nabothian cysts, and to note the presence or absence of a reddish "transformation zone" around the os *

• Performing a bimanual examination to check the angle and position of the cervix and uterus and to check for any pain or tenderness in the pelvic area

Most experienced practitioners say that they can eyeball the cervix while the speculum is in place and choose the best size with a high degree of accuracy. Dr. Koch prefers to measure the cervix during the speculum exam with an antique caliper. He says that this method, unique among cap fitters, is an accurate predictor of size and that he is able to choose the correct size almost every time. The caliper can take an accurate measure of the diameter of the cervix, but it cannot measure angle or symmetry, both of which strongly influence cap fit.

Inserting a cap into the vagina is similar to inserting a diaphragm and can be done by either the practitioner or by the woman herself. To insert the cap, fold it in half, then tip it into the vagina so that the mouth is facing toward the cervix, and guide it to the back by pushing on the rim with one or two fingers. (See pages 61–67 for more detailed information on insertion and removal.)

Sometimes fit is established with the first one or two cap insertions and others are simply tried for comparative purposes or to give a woman experience in insertion and removal. According to the Women's Health Service of Colorado Springs, occasionally a woman may need as many as fifteen insertions before she and her practitioner are satisfied that the fit is adequate. This case usually arises when a woman wants a cap very badly and fit is marginal.

The cervical cap fitting can be exciting and even liberating

---

* This area, also called the "squamo-columnar junction," normally covers the cervix in childhood and gradually retreats into the cervical canal as a woman matures. Sometimes it does not retreat all the way, leaving a reddish area around the os. This visible "transformation zone" is *perfectly normal*, but it is important to watch for any changes, because this spot seems to be more vulnerable to infection and the development of pre-cancerous conditions.

for many women, but a few find the session stressful and the visit can sometimes end in tears of frustration. If the cap fitting seems to be headed in this direction—and even if it is not—it is essential that practitioners de-emphasize performance and be supportive without being overbearing.

Even with the use of lubricating jelly the vaginal opening can become sore or irritated, and if this occurs, it is usually necessary to schedule a return visit to finish the fitting, or for further practice of insertion and removal. Because this problem is not always avoidable, it is very important to try to minimize the number of cap insertions to save a woman undue discomfort and extra clinic visits. At the initial cap fitting, women should be encouraged to return if they are unsure that the cap is staying on, or if they are experiencing cramping while the cap is in place.

Refit visits for the cervical cap are fairly common, but their frequency may vary quite a bit from practitioner to practitioner. In the Bernstein study, which encompassed eight clinical sites, the percentage of women who returned for at least one cap refit varied from 3.2 to 15.8. By comparison, diaphragm refits were substantially higher, varying from 16.7 to 40.9 percent. The report concludes that "those clinicians who fit a smaller portion of their [cap] subjects initially, refit far fewer of their clients."

WHEN DOES A CAP FIT?

There seems to be a general consensus that an ideally fit Prentif cavity rim cervical cap entirely covers the cervix, with its rim tucked snugly and evenly into the fornix (the conjunction of the vaginal walls and the cervix at the back of the vagina), that it has good suction, and that it cannot be easily dislodged by the fitter.

For most practitioners, the bottom line in acceptable fit is that no gaps exist between the rim and the cervix and that the cap cannot be easily dislodged by a reasonable amount of force. After the cap is in place, there are a number of maneuvers that can be performed to check fit:

• Make a full 360-degree sweep of the cap rim, searching for gaps or exposed parts of the cervix.

• If a gap is found, see if the rim pulls away easily.

• Using the notch at the base of the rim, try to rotate the cap. If it rotates easily, see if the cap tilts away from the cervix.

• After the cap has been in place for a minute or so, check the suction. Pinch the excess rubber of the dome between the tips of two fingers and tug. The dome should be collapsed. (This check is more difficult with the stiffer 22 mm and 25 mm sizes.)

• Although it is not possible to duplicate the activity of a vigorously thrusting penis in an office setting, the fitter should seek to dislodge the cap by pushing and tugging on it with one or two fingers from as many angles as possible, being careful not to hurt the woman.

It is essential to include each woman in an evaluation of her fit. She can offer her impression of how easy or difficult removal is for each size, how solid the suction appears to be, and, if two caps fit equally well, which one feels the most comfortable.

PROBLEMS IN CAP FITTING

Experienced cap fitters have identified several anatomical problems that can interfere with the fit of the Prentif cavity rim cap.

• If the cervix is quite long, the rim will not have contact with the fornix, and the cap will be more vulnerable to dislodgement.

• If the cervix is very short, the cap will not have enough of the neck to cling to and may be subject to being dislodged.

• If the cervix enters the vagina at an angle, one side of the cap will be exposed, making it more likely to be dislodged.

• If the cervix is shaped irregularly, either naturally or

from an obstetrical injury, the firm rim of the Prentif may not adhere to it securely.

• If the cap dome is not indented, it may mean that suction is not sufficient (except for the 22 mm size, which has little excess rubber to collapse).

CAP FIT

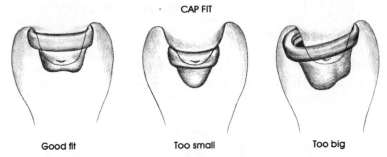

Good fit   Too small   Too big

The conditions above may be subtle or pronounced and more than one may exist. Hence, it is not always easy to say *why* a cap doesn't fit well. Nevertheless, many women want an explanation if they cannot be fit.

> **Note** All women need to be reassured that tipped uteruses; angled, asymmetrical cervixes, and long or short vaginas are completely within the range of normal body development and that failure to get a fit is most frequently an artifact of retarded technology rather than that something is wrong with them.

Most failures to get a good cap fit occur because the rigid rim of the Prentif does not conform to a cervix that is not relatively symmetrical and because there are not enough sizes to accommodate the wide variations in cervical anatomy.

One factor that has mystified many cap fitters is the propensity of certain caps to rotate easily on the cervix even if they appear to have good suction. Nurse Eileen Hatch, who fit caps in Ann Arbor, Michigan, under Dr. Johan Eliot's study, is unconcerned about rotation. "I had a 98 percent effectiveness rate and observed any number of caps that would rotate the entire 360 degrees. Perhaps rotation simply means that the cervix has room to swell a bit during sexual activity or during the last part of the cycle."

EXCELLENT FIT VERSUS ACCEPTABLE FIT

It is fair to say that cap investigators have agonized over cap fit more than any single issue. Most agree, however, that an ideal fit is one in which the cap covers the cervix completely, has a tight grip and strong suction, and is situated so that the rim is nestled snugly into the vaginal musculature surrounding the cervix.

Yet the matter of "adequate" fit remains a source of lively debate. Some experienced cap providers give ratings of 1, 2, and 3, or A, B, and C, to cap fit, while others use descriptive terms such as "excellent," "relative," "marginal," and "poor." If all of the conditions for fit are met, then the fit would be considered "excellent." If only some of the conditions are met but the cap appears to have good suction and cannot be readily dislodged with a finger, then the fit might be classified as "relative" or "marginal." In this case, a woman and her practitioner can evaluate the risks of getting pregnant in light of her immediate birth control needs, her contraceptive and health history, and her personal reasons for wanting a cap. If the fit is less than perfect, these circumstantial factors assume a magnified importance. Obvious gaps underneath the rim, poor suction, and ready dislodgement are all indicative of "poor" fit.

With full information about cap use and how to maximize its effectiveness with fertility awareness and backup during her fertile time, a highly motivated woman can make an informed decision about working with a less-than-perfect fit and might be able to use a cap effectively.

SMALL FIT VERSUS LARGE FIT

As can be seen from the chart on pages 192–196, a majority of the cervical cap investigators fit primarily sizes 22 and 25

Prentifs. Many of the practitioners find that the 22 seems to fit women who have never had children and say that they never or almost never fit a size 31. A significant minority, however, fit predominantly 28s with quite a few 25s and occasionally 31s and say that they rarely fit 22s. What does this discrepancy mean, if anything?

Masters and Johnson found that the uterus swells during sexual response. The cervix, by extension, may enlarge somewhat as well. Is it possible that smaller caps may sometimes pop off during orgasm, then become reattached as the resolution phase of sexual response occurs? Would a larger cap that takes more of the cervix into its dome stay on more securely during the dynamic changes of sexual response?

Ginny Cassidy-Brinn, a nurse practitioner and a director of the Los Angeles Feminist Women's Health Center, which always fit a large number of size 28 Prentifs, is baffled by the high number of 22s that many practitioners fit. "I wonder," she says, "if they are fitting the cervical cap or the cervical beanie."

Another puzzling issue relating to fit is whether or not the cap's rim, which may be buried snugly in the fornix at the fitting, is exposed during sexual response when the vagina balloons out and the uterus is pulled back. If this is the case, should women who have all or part of the rim exposed at the time of their fitting be automatically disqualified for cap use? With the exception of the work of Masters and Johnson, no one has considered what happens to the cervix and uterus during sexual response, but accurate information on this subject could affect cap fit and future designs.

Women can be confused about controversies over fitting and it can influence their confidence in the cap. Nevertheless, it is probably best to be honest about unknowns. "I explain to women that we don't have a chance to do 'field testing' on the cap and that they need to use a backup method until they are confident it is staying in place during intercourse," Eileen Hatch says.

WHO CAN BE FIT?

The chart on pages 192–196 reveals that practitioners fit widely varying percentages of women who ask for caps. Some of the variation in fitting rates can be attributed to the underlying goals of the different investigators participating in the FDA study. Some set out to produce an excellent effectiveness rate and therefore fit mostly women who had extremely secure fits. Others wanted to provide caps to large numbers of women who have few viable contraceptive options, and let many women with relative or marginal fits try to use the cap. In many cases, their effectiveness rates were as good as some very highly controlled studies. Fit rates varied from a low of 30 percent at the Vermont Feminist Health Center in Burlington to a high of 90 percent at some clinics, with a majority falling between 60 and 80 percent. It is interesting to note that the Vermont clinic has a 91.5 percent use-effectiveness rate, the same as many practitioners who fit a much higher percentage of women. These profoundly inharmonious figures raise some intriguing questions that are likely to be debated for some time.

• Is there a golden mean somewhere between fitting almost everybody and fitting almost nobody?
• What are acceptable minimal fitting standards?
• Why do some women who have excellent fits and who use the cap consistently and correctly still get pregnant?
• When fitting rates vary so widely, how can effectiveness rates be so similar?
• How important is the use of spermicide?
• How can different practitioners have different fitting criteria but similar effectiveness rates and, conversely, similar fitting criteria and different effectiveness rates?
• Just how important is fit, anyway?

These questions and many others regarding fit need to be investigated in the immediate future, using the Prentif as well as other existing and experimental models, to broaden our concept of appropriate fitting standards.

IS THERE AN IDEAL TIME TO FIT THE CAP?

The cap can be fit at any point in the menstrual cycle, including during the menstrual period, if the flow is not so heavy that it inhibits a woman or practitioner from freely participating in the fitting. Women are frequently embarrassed or uncomfortable about being fit during days of heavy menstrual flow, but it should not necessarily affect cap fit. Some practitioners prefer to fit the cap around midcycle, between day 10 and day 18 of a regular monthly cycle, thereby avoiding menstruation.

Nurse Practitioner Renee Potik asks women who have been on the Pill to discontinue for two months before getting a cap fitting because "on the Pill, the cervix does not undergo normal hormonally stimulated changes, so the fit might not be accurate." Eileen Hatch reports that she occasionally has to do refits on women who were fit while they were taking the Pill. "They would notice cramping or a tightness at midcycle, or just feel like the cap didn't fit well," she says. Most practitioners see a few women who actually need two different size caps, because they have such severe edema (swelling from fluid retention) during the latter part of their cycles.

TRAINING CAP USERS

The first time you insert your own cervical cap, you will not be able to tell whether it is on the cervix or not. You may feel inadequate, clumsy, or embarrassed, but it happens to everyone. If the cap becomes attached to the vaginal wall, instead of removing it altogether, it is often possible for your practitioner to break the suction and coax it onto the cervix. Then you can see what a correctly placed cap feels like.

A trick Dr. Koch uses in checking insertion technique is to surreptitiously displace the cap and ask each woman to check it for herself. If she thinks the cap is in place, he insists on further instruction and practice.

If you have had diaphragm experience, you may adapt to cap insertion and removal after just a few tries. If you have problems initially, you will usually be able to overcome them with a strong desire to use the cap and with encouragement from your practitioner.

THE CONFIDENCE FACTOR

Cap investigators have puzzled over fit, worried about dislodgements, and wondered about the absolute necessity of spermicide. Yet quite a number mention that some women have discontinued cap use because of a "lack of confidence" that the cap will protect them from pregnancy, occasionally noting a male partner's lack of confidence as well. Generally, from 1 to 5 percent of women who discontinue cap use do so because they have doubts about effectiveness.

Dr. Johan Eliot, who coordinated an eight-site cap study in Michigan and Ohio, has systematically explored numerous facets of cap use and concluded that "the single strongest predictor [of satisfaction and continuation] was confidence in the cap."

Eliot's conceptual model of satisfaction, continuation, and effectiveness, published in the *Journal of Reproductive Medicine*,* is a thought-provoking analysis of the effect of confidence on continued use of the cap and, ultimately, on its effectiveness.

This concept illustrates that good cap fit is only one factor in effectiveness. It is clear that there is an elaborate host of factors that impinge upon proper and continued use from the user's point of view, and their rank and importance may vary quite a bit from woman to woman. One element that the model does not explore is that of practitioner attitude and commitment to user education and support. This component, as noted in the discussion of practitioner bias on pages 99 to

* Johan Eliot, Leslie Anderson, and Stan Bernstein, "Progress Report on a Study of the Cervical Cap," *Journal of Reproductive Medicine* 30 (10), Oct. 1985, p. 756.

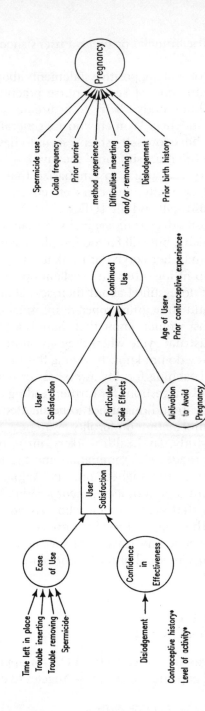

Conceptual model of contraceptive cap satisfaction, continuation and effectiveness

1a) Satisfaction

Time left in place
Trouble inserting*
Trouble removing*
Spermicide

Ease of Use

User Satisfaction

Dislodgement

Confidence in Effectiveness

Contraceptive history*
Level of activity*

*These variables are expected to condition the effects of all of the other predictors.

1b) Continuation

User Satisfaction

Particular Side Effects

Motivation to Avoid Pregnancy

Continued Use*

Age of User*
Prior contraceptive experience*

*These variables are expected to condition the effects of all of the other predictors.

1c) Effectiveness

Spermicide use
Coital frequency
Prior barrier
method experience
Difficulties inserting
and/or removing cap
Dislodgement
Prior birth history

Pregnancy

101 can be critical and can make or break a user's successful use of any method.

"We make a point of making positive statements about the cap," says Rose Heman, one of several nurse practitioners who participated in Eliot's study. "I try to assure all women that practice builds confidence. Women who are generally not sure of themselves, or have low self-esteem, seem to have the hardest time and need the most support," she says.

It can also be very reassuring to emphasize that when used consistently and correctly, the cap's effectiveness can approach that of the mini-pill and the IUD.

Feminists have been advocating vaginal self-examination for more than fifteen years, but still far too few physicians take the time to show a woman her cervix, or think it is important to do so. A cervical cap fitting offers an excellent opportunity for women to become demystified about their sexual and reproductive anatomy and to acquire *concrete* information on fertility awareness. Most women know that there is a time in the middle of the menstrual cycle when they are more likely to get pregnant, but they do not know how long this time lasts or how to identify it. Teaching fertility awareness or handing out written material and suggestions for further reading is vital to effective use of the cap and ought not to be slighted. (See page 154 for detailed information on fertility awareness.)

During the FDA study, lay health workers, nurse practitioners, and midwives made self-examination and the teaching of fertility awareness the highest priority. While such information is important in and of itself, incorporating it into the cap fitting assures that even women who can not be fit with a cap don't leave their appointment empty-handed. They gain positive self-knowledge and leave with specific information on how to make any method of birth control more effective.

THE IMPORTANCE OF PRACTITIONER TRAINING

Even before the cap was submitted to the FDA for approval, a group of experienced cap fitters met in Los Angeles to design a comprehensive training program for prospective cap providers. Their goal was to be ready to train new cap practitioners quickly and effectively, both before approval and immediately after, so that the many women who seek caps have a good chance of receiving competent, efficient care, even though many practitioners may be new and relatively inexperienced. This group plans to offer training seminars around the country and to provide on-site training for individual practitioners who are unable to attend the seminars. Information on this program can be obtained from the National Women's Health Network at 202/543-9222.

A program of this type seems essential to acceptance of the cap by women and their partners, as well as by the medical community. The demise of Dr. Foote's cap one hundred years ago because of the widespread reproduction of poor quality caps and, one might assume, incompetent provision, illustrates the urgent necessity for the highest standards of cap provision from the very beginning of its new lease on life.

5 ✳ SELECTING A PRACTITIONER
and Seeking a Second Opinion

Even though gynecologists and birth control clinics tend to favor the Pill, most also provide diaphragms. But in the first few years after it is approved in the United States, the cervical cap will not be universally available, and it may be difficult to find a provider in some areas of the country. Even after finding where you can obtain a cap, you may encounter practitioners who are ambivalent about its use or are not very experienced fitters. But don't be discouraged. Many family-planning clinics and other medical practitioners will be eager to offer a new, low-risk birth control alternative, especially one that has demonstrated excellent potential in so many recent studies.

WHO WILL PROVIDE CERVICAL CAPS?

Undoubtedly most of the investigators who offered caps before and during the FDA study will continue to fit them. This group (refer to page 185) includes feminist clinics, state and locally funded family-planning clinics, physicians, nurse practitioners, physicians' assistants, and midwives. By now many of these practitioners have seven or eight years of experience in fitting cervical caps and would be excellent choices, if they are within driving distance. It is also a good idea to call your own gynecologist or family doctor since she or he may well offer cervical caps; if you are a regular patient, it should be easy to get an appointment.

There are 700 Planned Parenthood offices nationwide which offer referrals for birth control and abortion and 190 affiliates which provide birth control services. After it is approved by the FDA, all Planned Parenthood clinics will offer the cap as a regular part of their birth control services. Planned Parenthood clinics and offices can be easily located through the telephone book or through Directory Assistance.

Many abortion clinics also provide birth control services and quite a number will certainly begin dispensing cervical caps as well. These clinics advertise heavily, especially in the Yellow Pages. Check under "Abortion," "Birth Control," "Clinics," or "Health Clinics" in the Yellow Pages for listings of such facilities in your area. Federally, state, and locally funded family-planning clinics, where birth control services are usually the least expensive, can be found in the Yellow Pages under the same headings.

Many nurse practitioners, physicians' assistants, and midwives have their own practices and many will certainly offer cervical caps, but because of state and local regulations, these practitioners frequently work in clinics or are attached to established physicians' practices and may not be listed separately in the White or Yellow Pages. Some do have their own practices and advertise separately, especially in neighborhood and alternative newspapers which frequently carry ads and listings of womens' health services.

MAKING AN APPOINTMENT

When shopping around for a practitioner who fits cervical caps, it is best to get as much information as you can over the phone, because practices vary widely. Since caps are so new, and standards for their provision will probably vary widely, it might be wise to ask some questions over the phone when making an appointment so that you will have a clear idea about what kind of service you will be getting and so that you can ascertain the practitioner's attitude toward the cap. Don't be afraid to ask:

• How long does the fitting usually take, and will you be allowed extra time if you need it?

• Who will be doing the fitting—M.D., nurse practitioner, physicians' assistant, midwife, or lay health worker—and what kind of training and experience do they have?

• What is the price and are there any extra charges for a Pap smear or other lab work?

• Is a follow-up visit required, and if so is there a charge for it?

• What percentage of women are fit?

• What is the cost of the visit if you are not able to be fit or decide not to get a cap?

• Will an experienced staff member be available to answer questions by phone if you have an urgent question before your follow-up visit?

• Is it possible for your partner to attend the cap fitting with you?

• Are there any restrictions on who can get a cap—such as age, contraceptive experience, or abortion history?

If the receptionist can't answer your questions, you might ask to speak to a nurse or someone who works closely with caps and ask the questions that seem most important to you. If you live in a large or medium-sized city, you might choose to contact several cap fitters and get as much of the previously outlined information as possible before deciding which one to see. Family planning and feminist clinics are usually very helpful on the phone, but busy doctors' offices may be unwilling to give out such detailed information prior to an office visit.

SEEKING A SECOND OPINION

Experienced cap practitioners agree on many things, such as the need for detailed instructions on cap use and the importance of letting each woman see her cervix before the cap fitting. They do not agree on who can be fit for a cervical cap. The wide variation in fitting rates (see chart on pages 192–196) suggests that if you are told you cannot be fit by one practitioner, you may have a very good chance of being successfully fit by another.

If you have been told you can't be fit by one practitioner, it might be useful to do some "market research" before making another appointment. If you live in a medium-sized or large city, you can probably find several clinics or physicians who fit caps. In this case, call and ask what percentage of women each fits. If rates vary quite a bit, your best bet is probably to choose the one who fits the most women. If you live in a small town, this choice may not be available to you and you might have to wait until you take a vacation, or plan a trip to a larger city.

It is very important to be completely honest with practitioners with any relevant information concerning your visit, but when seeking a second opinion on cap fit, it might be a good idea not to mention your other visit until the end of your appointment, so that you can get a completely unbiased opinion. After the fitting, you can discuss aspects of both fittings and better evaluate your fit. If both practitioners express the same opinion about your fit, then you might have to give up on the Prentif for now. If their reasons are clearly conflicting you might want to get yet another opinion. If you are really determined to get a cap, you can try to locate a practitioner who fits the Dumas cap on an experimental basis. Although the National Women's Health Network does not make referrals, it maintains a listing of many cap providers and may be able to offer tips on tracking down a provider who fits the Dumas. The Network, located in Washington, D.C., can be reached at (202) 543-9222.

WHAT IF YOU CAN'T BE FIT?

If after getting a second opinion you simply cannot be fit, or you have a contraindication to cap use, you may want to discuss other birth control options with your practitioner. Chapter 11, "A Comprehensive Survey of Birth Control Options," offers an overview of the available methods in a format designed to help you compare the various alternatives. If you have already tried the most obvious methods, you might want to try some inventive combinations of less widely used methods—which can be highly effective if practiced faithfully.

A failure to get fit with a cervical cap can be very disappointing, but it is impossible to tell beforehand whether or not one of the available sizes will be right for you. Therefore, it is a good idea to go to the fitting armed with the knowledge that not everyone *can* wear the Prentif, and be prepared to investigate alternatives.

6 ✳ AT HOME WITH YOUR CAP:
Step-by-Step Information on Use and Care

One of the most delightful aspects of getting a cervical cap is the opportunity it offers many women for self-discovery and increased knowledge about a part of their bodies that has heretofore been the sole province of the gynecologist. "My cervix always seemed as remote as my gallbladder," says a college student from San Diego. "What a surprise when I found that it was literally at my fingertip."

Becoming familiar with the angle and location of your cervix is essential for insertion and removal of the cervical cap, as well as for checking placement before and after intercourse. Your practitioner should let you see your cervix with the speculum in place and help you practice locating it manually as well.

Before you insert the cap, feel for your cervix with your index finger. Some women say that they can just reach it with a fingertip, but most can feel it readily as a firm knob and can make out the indentation in the center which is the os, or opening to the cervical canal. Insert a finger as far as you can into your vagina and move your fingertip around. The cervix feels firm but pliant, somewhat like the end of your nose. If you have a hard time finding it, bear down like you are trying to have a hard bowel movement. This will help push both the cervix and the cap a little closer toward your finger. Practice until you are sure of what you are feeling. A few women with quite long vaginas and/or short fingers may have difficulty in feeling the cervix, but most can locate it readily.

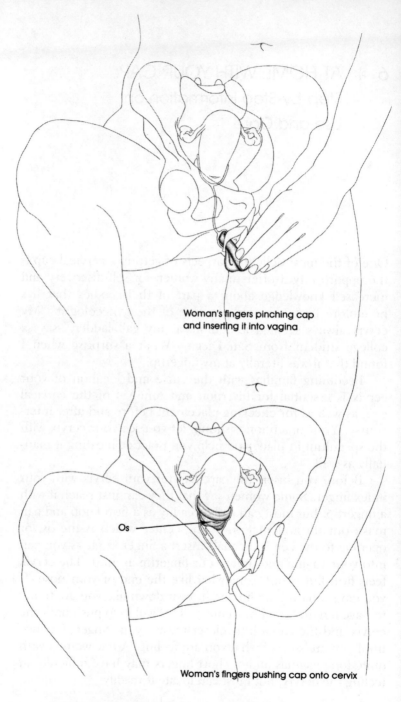

Woman's fingers pinching cap
and inserting it into vagina

Os

Woman's fingers pushing cap onto cervix

The rectum runs parallel to the length of the vagina and sometimes, if you have not had a recent bowel movement, you can feel feces through the vaginal wall and mistake their firmness for the cervix. After a few weeks, though, you should be able to make the distinctions between vaginal walls, the firm, smooth cervix, and hard, lumpy feces.

INSERTION

Most women find that lying down or reclining on a few pillows is the most comfortable position for insertion and removal of the cervical cap, but others prefer to squat or stand with one foot on a chair or the side of the bathtub. (A lot of women routinely remove the cap in the shower, standing in a slightly bent-over position.)

Inserting the cervical cap consists of two simple steps: *getting the cap into the vagina* and *placing it on the cervix.* After filling the cap about one third to one half full with spermicide, pinch the rim firmly and ease it into the vagina, tipping the cap so that the mouth or open part is facing toward the back. (Information on spermicide use appears on page 68.) As soon as the cap is inside, deliberately push the rim to the back with one or two fingers, visualizing where the cervix is and aiming for that spot. The vaginal canal is not open and empty. The folded, fleshy mucous membrane walls touch each other, filling the vagina up, something like rolls of wet cotton in a tube. You can't just slip the cap in and expect it to segue back to the cervix. You have to purposefully push it past two or three inches of puffy vaginal tissue.

> **Note** When driving a car through sand or soft mud, the rule is that once you start, you must keep going or risk getting stuck. This rule applies to cap insertion as well. If you stop pushing it too soon it may settle onto the vaginal wall.

The suction can be strong and you might think that the cap is in place. So, be aggressive. When the cap gets in the vicinity of the cervix, it should go on easily. Most women don't feel anything as it slips on, but a few detect faint sensations of the cap taking hold. "Sometimes I feel a little tug on my uterus as the cap slips on. Then I know it is in place," a long-time cap user from Los Angeles says.

Now check to see if the cap is in place. If it is, you should be able to feel only the cap dome and the rim. Search thoroughly around the rim to make sure that the cervix isn't camped beside it. Try to feel the firm cervix through the dome. If you are using a larger cap (28 or 31) the dome should be collapsed, and you may be able to feel the cervix through the rubber. The rubber on the 22s and 25s is slightly firmer than on the larger sizes, which makes it more difficult to distinguish anything through it. If you are not sure the cap is in place, take it out, locate the cervix with your finger, and try again.

Note The back of the vagina is a blind alley, or cul-de-sac, sealed off so that nothing—caps, sponges, tampons —can get lost. The only opening is the os, where menstrual blood and cervical secretions come out. The os is also the gateway for sperm, which must be protected by the cervical cap.

WHEN TO INSERT THE CAP

Since the cap can be worn for several days or even a week at a time, you can insert it at your convenience, depending upon your personal tastes and habits. Some women use the cap like the diaphragm, inserting it only if they are planning to have sex and removing it six to eight hours later. Others like the convenience of being able to put it in when they shower in the morning and forget about it until they are ready to remove it.

Many practitioners recommend that the cap be inserted

> **Note** No matter what your pattern of use is, the cap, like the diaphragm, should remain in place for six to eight hours after your last session of intercourse.

at least one-half hour ahead of intercourse, so that "the suction can build up." This recommendation is based upon the assumption that the suction becomes stronger over time. But there is no evidence upon which to base this conclusion. Dr. Koch, who has studied the biomechanics of cap fit in detail, points out that the device stays on by a combination of suction and gripping which is active as soon as the cap is in place. Many women have been baffled by the requirement and report that they ignore it anyway. "Waiting a half hour after insertion to have intercourse requires a considerable degree of forethought—that's no improvement over the diaphragm," says one Brooklyn, New York, social worker who has used the cap for about two years.

Even though you can insert the cap well ahead of intercourse, it is okay to put it in immediately before sex as well. But if you wait until you are very aroused you may have trouble with insertion because the urethral sponge—the ridge of erectile tissue that runs along the roof of the vagina— becomes very firm when engorged with blood during sexual response and the vaginal walls puff up and become much denser. Experienced cap users have probably encountered this problem more than once and have discovered the limits of what they can and cannot do, but new users might be concerned that something is wrong with their insertion technique. It's a good idea to keep some condoms handy for instances such as this. If you find that this situation arises frequently, try putting the cap in either in the morning before work or school, before dinner, or before going out, *even if you are unsure about what the evening may bring*. Unlike the diaphragm, which can drip and become uncomfortable after several hours, the cap will remain neatly and unobtrusively in place for as long as you want to leave it.

An Atlanta student discovered another problem associ-

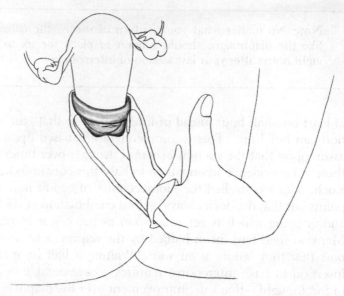

Woman's finger touching cervix through dome of cap

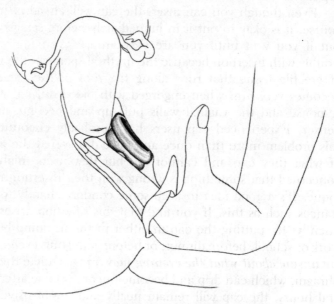

Misplaced cap with woman's fingers feeling cervix

ated with last-minute insertion. "I never had trouble with insertion except once when I was inebriated," she says. "We were laughing a lot and I just couldn't get it in, so we had to use a condom." Minor problems like this are typical at first, or might occur occasionally when you have intercourse unexpectedly, but they are rarely a problem for experienced cap users.

REMOVAL

Some women can easily remove their caps while lying down, but others find squatting, kneeling, or putting a foot up on a chair is helpful. Many women have found that sitting on the toilet can help when nothing else will. This position allows the muscles to relax more and lets the uterus move forward so that the rim of the cap is easier to reach.

The standard way to remove the cap is to press on the rim with a finger until the suction is broken, so that you can tilt it off the cervix. If you have very short fingers or a long vagina, this technique may not work and you may have to resort to some of the tricks listed on page 73. With the larger caps, it is often possible to grasp the dome with a finger and thumb and coax both the cervix and cap forward a little so that the rim is more accessible. Since the uterus is suspended on ligaments which are slightly elastic, it is somewhat mobile, and you can pull it forward a bit without fear of hurting yourself or straining the ligaments. Once you have successfully broken the suction, ease your fingertip over the rim and inside of the cap and pull it out sideways.

On occasion, no matter what you do, a stubborn cap may not come off. If you have tried everything, simply forget about it for a while. Often the uterus has just retreated slightly and moved the cap rim just out of reach. It will return to its normal position when you are more relaxed and you can try again.

Removal is not an enduring problem for most women, but it can be a little more difficult than insertion, especially at first. Women and their practitioners have developed quite a number of self-help techniques to help overcome removal dif-

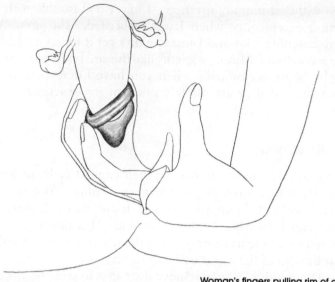

Woman's fingers pulling rim of cap
to break suction for removal

ficulties. (If you have continuing difficulties with removal, turn to "Tricks to Help with Removal" on page 73 for more information.)

With a basic understanding of vaginal anatomy and a few tips on insertion and removal, most women learn to use the cervical cap quickly and easily. After a few months, as its use becomes routine, new cap users gain confidence in its effectiveness and appreciate the freedom that it affords.

PARTNER ASSISTANCE

Some women who have good communication with their partners have successfully taught them to help with insertion or removal and have incorporated this utilitarian detail into their sexual routine. If you don't have enough information or confidence to teach your partner adequately, call your practitioner and see if it would be possible for you both to go in for a follow-up visit. Partners who have learned insertion and removal techniques can also take responsibility for checking cap placement both before and after intercourse, either routinely, or once in a while if you are not sure it is on the cervix.

While the majority of men don't give birth control much thought, many are pleased to be able to share in the responsibility and take it very seriously. If you have a cap or are thinking about getting one and have a steady partner, getting him to read this book might be very helpful.

HOW LONG CAN THE CAP BE LEFT IN PLACE?

There are several standards for the length of time the cap may be kept in place. Since the early 1970s, the patient instructions that accompany Lamberts' caps have recommended leaving them in place for "no more than about 24 hours in all." But practitioners in the United States and Canada generally feel that this recommendation is excessively conservative for the Prentif and Dumas and nullifies one of the cap's most desirable attributes; that is, inserting it and not having to think about it again for a few days. The majority of practitioners recommend keeping the cap in place for no more than three days, not because of potential health problems, but because of an observed "odor threshold."

Note Because of concerns about Toxic Shock Syndrome, many practitioners suggest that the cap and diaphragm not be worn during menstrual bleeding. Others think it is okay as long as you insert it just before intercourse and remove it promptly six to eight hours afterward.

Yet many of the thirty-five hundred women in Dr. Koch's study have worn the cap up to seven days without adverse effects. The Federation of Feminist Women's Health Centers clinics suggest that women adjust cap wear to fit their individual needs, taking into consideration the frequency of sexual activity, health history, and current vaginal conditions. The chart on page 192–196 shows variations in the *average* length of wear for women in more than sixty studies.

If you are having sex only infrequently, you might choose to use the cap like the diaphragm, changing it daily. If you have sex frequently during the week and several times on the weekend, you may want to remove it less often.

USE OF SPERMICIDE

The standard recommendation for using spermicide with the cap is to place from a teaspoon to a tablespoon of spermicidal cream or jelly inside of the dome, so that it is about one third to one half full. There seems to be general agreement among U.S. and Canadian providers that no additional spermicide should be put on the rim, as is recommended with the diaphragm, although some may get there anyway during insertion. The patient package insert that comes with the Prentif advises using additional spermicide if you have intercourse after the cap has been in place for a few hours, but this seems totally unnecessary and, some practitioners feel, may actually interfere with the cap's suction.

Based on the results of the 1953 study by Tietze, Lehfeldt, and Liebmann on spermicide use with the hard plastic cap, nearly all U.S. cap investigators recommend the use of spermicide. Otherwise, there is little hard data on the subject. The chart on pages 192–196 shows few studies in which all women used spermicide 100 percent of the time. Most women do use it consistently, but some use it only during their fertile times, while a few use it infrequently or not at all. Some women who have allergies to the chemicals in commercial spermicides make their own out of lemon juice and aloe vera gel, or just use plain lemon juice inside of the cap.

Linda Stein, a nurse practitioner at the Alternative Health Center in Seattle, is one of the few practitioners who has addressed the issue of effectiveness and spermicide use directly. Her report to the FDA including use of both Prentif and Dumas caps indicates that 30 percent of the eight hundred women in her study always used spermicide, 23 percent sometimes used it, and 47 percent never used it. However, the use-effectiveness for both caps was 83.5 percent, somewhat lower than many of the studies in which women used spermicide consistently.

Dr. Bernstein evaluated the contents of the caps and the cervical canals of ten women who used spermicide and left their devices in for three days. Viable sperm were found in one cap, but the concentration was probably not high enough to result in pregnancy. This study is far too small to be conclusive and needs to be redone, examining caps and the cervical mucus both with and without the use of spermicide.

In 1961, Drs. Lehfeldt, Sobrero, and Inglis published the results of a study they did investigating the effectiveness of spermicidal cream and jelly for long-term cap use. They found active ingredients from cream preparations inside the cap at the end of five days, but none for the jelly, and concluded that the water-soluble jelly breaks down faster than the cream. On the basis of this study, most cap practitioners recommend the use of spermicidal *cream* if the cap is going to be kept in for three days or longer.

DOES SPERMICIDE HAVE HARMFUL EFFECTS?

Until 1982, no one had questioned the safety of spermicidal cream or jelly. Then a study was published, suggesting a possible association between the use of vaginal spermicides and birth defects.* The report received national attention and as is common in such situations, the essential facts became badly distorted in the public mind. When hard questions were raised, the researchers admitted that their data was only suggestive.†

A good bit of spermicide does pass through the highly

---

* H. Jick, A. M. Walker, and K. J. Rothman, et al, "Vaginal Spermicides and Congenital Disorders," *Journal of the American Medical Association* 245 (1981), p. 1329.

† Richard N. Watkins, one of the co-authors of this study, recently published a letter in the *Journal of the American Medical Association* (Dec. 12, 1986) repudiating the study's methodology and conclusions. He wrote: "These data indicate that our study's definition of exposure to spermicide near the time of conception was grossly inaccurate and that its conclusion is unsupported by more complete evidence from its subjects."

absorbent vaginal walls and enters the bloodstream, but much of it is probably broken down by the liver and excreted in the urine, although some may be absorbed by certain body tissues. At this point, much more investigation needs to be done.

In regard to spermicides, the cervical cap has several advantages over the diaphragm. With the diaphragm a wide expanse of highly absorbent mucous membrane is exposed to the spermicide. But with the cap, because the spermicide stays in the dome and you don't have to add any extra for repeated intercourse, it is far less messy and a much smaller area of the *less absorbent cervical surface* is in contact with the cream or jelly. Thus, there is far less that can be absorbed. An added benefit of the cap is that over a year's time, the average woman will use about one tenth as much spermicide with the cap as with the diaphragm, making the cap far cheaper than the diaphragm.

CARE OF THE CAP

Care of the cervical cap is quite similar to that of the diaphragm. Wash it with soap and water and keep it away from excessive heat or cold. Many practitioners suggest drying the cap and powdering it with cornstarch—which absorbs oils and helps preserve the rubber—and storing it in some sort of container. Unlike diaphragms, caps do not come in durable carrying cases, so you may want to find one of your own. Little plastic boxes like the ones carried in novelty stores are perfect for this purpose. Sturdy containers are also recommended since it is rumored that well-seasoned cervical caps are a favorite play-toy of cats.

If you want to deodorize your cap, don't boil it, because the heat will cause the rubber to deteriorate. Try some of the inventive home remedies listed on pages 82–83 instead. Be careful of cold as well. One woman left her cap to air out on the windowsill on a cold Vermont night and found it the next morning, cracked in half! Occasionally, when you are cleaning your cap, it is a good idea to check for holes, cracks, or wear. Also watch for weak or thin spots on the dome. Fill the dome with water and look for any pinhole leaks. If your cap is starting to look badly worn, think about getting a new one. Most Prentif caps will last from one to three years; some considerably longer, depending on the amount of use and the kind of care they get.

7 ✳ STUMBLING BLOCKS WITH THE PRENTIF CAP:
Solutions and Alternatives

The side effects of the cap seem likely to constitute annoyances to users, rather than threats to their lives or health.

—Dr. James P. Koch
Contraception
February 1982

Compared to the lengthy catalog of disorders that can be caused by use of synthetic hormones or intrauterine devices, the problems that occur with the Prentif cavity rim cervical cap are minor indeed. Of the scant handful of problems that have been identified with use of the Prentif, none threaten life or health, none negatively affect future fertility, and most of them have turned out to be remarkably similar to the problems that have been reported over the years by diaphragm users.

DIFFICULTIES WITH INSERTION OR REMOVAL

One of the most persistent myths about the cervical cap is that it is difficult to insert and remove. Often this alleged drawback to the cap is put in terms of "more difficult than the diaphragm," with an open-ended implication about the frequency and degree of difficulty, leaving the impression that insertion and removal are "hurdles" that new users must overcome. In real life, most women, especially those with diaphragm experience, do not have any trouble at all after practicing as little as two or three times. "I can't believe how easy this is" is a comment that practitioners hear over and over.

Nevertheless, a small percentage of women do have some difficulty, at least at first, either because they have not had diaphragm experience, or because they have an unfortunate combination of short fingers and a long vagina. The few women who are genuinely squeamish or timid about handling their own genitals may experience some difficulties. There are also a few women who don't have any specific problems, but who never seem to develop a "feel" for the cap, or confidence in their insertion techniques. (See page 50 for information on the importance of confidence in cap effectiveness.)

The most helpful solution to uncertainties about insertion or difficulties with removal is commitment on the part of the user and patience and·support from the practitioner. In some cases, several follow-up visits in the first few weeks of cap use may be necessary to help a few women acquire confidence in their insertion and removal skills. "I was never sure I was getting the cap in the right place," an Atlanta cap user reports. "So I went back to the clinic for a refresher course. After that, I was fine." Like this woman, if you are uncertain about any aspect of cap use, even after one follow-up visit, don't be embarrassed or feel inadequate. Call your practitioner and go back for a refit, a check of your insertion skills, and an evaluation of your cap experience. If you otherwise like your cap and have no viable choice among other available birth control methods, the time spent in solving problems may be well worth it.

TRICKS TO HELP WITH REMOVAL

In the past, many of the European cervical caps came with strings already attached, and both the Prentif and the Vimule are designed to be used with them. The little notch at the base of the Prentif's rim is in fact intended to have a string attached.

To put a string on your cap, take a darning needle and work it through the notch or cap rim, then pull a length of heavy dental floss, fishing line, or synthetic string through, making a loop about an inch or two in length. Use the same hole for successive strings.

A loop can be quite helpful in coaxing the rim of the cap closer to the front of the vagina so that you can get better leverage on it with your finger. If you have strong suction, tugging on a string will not necessarily pull the cap off the cervix, but it should help bring the rim within easier reach. Some women have their partners help with insertion or removal, either on a regular basis or occasionally, but many women do not have this option. (See page 66 for more information on partner assistance.)

If fingers, strings, or partners don't work, you might consider using an instrument to aid cap removal. If your first response to this is negative, consider this: speculums, both

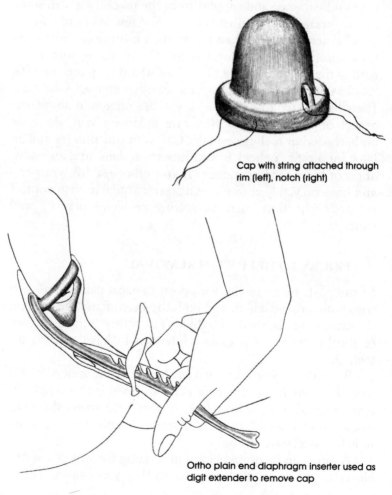

Cap with string attached through rim (left), notch (right)

Ortho plain end diaphragm inserter used as digit extender to remove cap plastic and metal, are occasionally inserted into the vagina. So are plastic inserters for tampons, spermicides and medications, douche nozzles—maybe even dildos and those plastic diaphragm inserters that never seem to work.

If you happen to have an old diaphragm inserter tucked away in your drawer, consider it for new use. Several Los Angeles cap users report using this inserter successfully as a "digit extender" by pressing the finger against the shaft about an inch or so below the flat end and then pressing the end against the cap rim.

Ortho used to make an inserter/remover with a hooked end similar to a giant plastic crochet hook. One New York print-shop owner who had quite a bit of trouble with removal used one of these inserters and found it very useful.

"At first, you don't know what you are doing, but you soon get a sense about how far in the tip of the inserter needs to go. I guide the hook up the side of the cap until I think it is in far enough and then turn it so that the hook will engage the edge of the rim, then slowly pull it out. Sometimes, after I break the suction, the cap will come off, but slip back on, so I have to try again."

Ortho has stopped making the hooked inserters, but the ones with the plain end can usually be purchased at a pharmacy. If the pharmacist will not give you one without a prescription, ask your cap fitter to write one for you. Remember also that clinics can order diaphragm inserters from Ortho in bulk, so that they are available during cap fittings for women who have initial difficulties with removal.

USER DISCOMFORT

Women who use diaphragms frequently report cramps, discomfort, or even pain after wearing the device for the required six to eight hours, and many who decide to switch to the cap continually marvel at how comfortable it is. Most women find that once the cap is in place they cannot feel it at all and are able to completely forget that it is there. A small percentage of women, however, report experiencing "an undefined creepy sensation," "pressure," "tightness," or "vague cramping," at least some of the time, or from extended cap wear. A very few say that they feel pressure on the bladder or rectum, as many diaphragm users do, but almost no one stops using the cap because of these minor physical sensations.

Researchers who have studied the mechanics of cap stability are in general agreement that the Prentif stays on the cervix through a combination of gripping and suction. If this is indeed the case, then it is no surprise that some cramping might result, especially with the smaller caps favored by many practitioners.

A few women say that they can feel the cap during intercourse, with sensations ranging from "mild" to "somewhat distracting," and occasionally "fairly severe." One woman describes experiencing "the sensation of a solid object being pushed into the vaginal wall." Once in a while women report to their practitioners that they stopped using the cap because it was painful during intercourse. Some women have found that avoiding specific sexual positions will eliminate discomfort and that this alteration is not a very big sacrifice to make for the comfort gained. Others have discovered that discomfort only occurs at certain times during the cycle and use an alternate method if the sensations are strong enough to be distracting.

A small number of women have found that using a larger cap between ovulation and the onset of menses alleviates cramping or feelings of tightness that may be caused by premenstrual fluid retention. If you notice that discomfort or dislodgements are occurring during the last part of your cycle, you might want to schedule a refit appointment during that time.

PARTNER DISCOMFORT

From 10 to 15 percent of cap users mention that their partners feel the firm rim of the Prentif during intercourse and some discontinue cap use for this reason. In the Los Angeles Cervical Cap Study, partner complaints accounted for 11 percent of the cap discontinuations, but the study notes that "some women specify that their partners do not complain"—rather, they "notice that the cap is there." Some men report that they can feel the cap "sometimes" or "at certain angles." One Florida newspaper editor found that the cap pinched his penis and was "as hard as a rock." He says, "We had to keep shifting around to avoid it, but eventually found that there were certain positions that were more comfortable."

"Most men can't feel it at all," a Brooklyn, New York, sex therapist told her practitioner. "But one boyfriend said that his penis would hit against the hard rubber of the rim and that it hurt him."

In addition to discomfort caused by the rim of the Prentif, partners report an occasional scratch or abrasion on the penis, and the notch, which may be used to attach a string, has been identified as the most likely culprit. Similar minor injuries can also occur with the diaphragm and the IUD, which sometimes causes scratches on the penis from its stiff plastic strings. One woman notes that the raised lettering on the curved rim of the Vimule irritated her partner's penis. "I removed it with an emery board," she says. "It took a long time, but it worked." The notch can also be snipped off with sharp fingernail scissors or a razor blade, then the rough "scar" can be smoothed with an emery board.

Dealing with partner discomfort varies greatly, depending as much on how assertive a woman feels she can be about her own needs in sex as on how severe the discomfort is. Some women stop using the cap at the slightest complaint from their partners, while others stand their ground and insist that men assume some of the unwanted physical effects that seem to be part and parcel of many birth control methods. One woman reports that when her boyfriend complained that he could "feel" the cap, she thought, "If that's all he has to put up with for me to be safe, I figure it's okay."

"I caution women not to bring up the subject of partner discomfort until something happens—it's just too risky," says Nurse Practitioner Eileen Hatch. "Some men will object to the slightest inconvenience." This seems to be sound advice, but if your partner exhibits signs of obvious discomfort or gets a scratch or abrasion on his penis, then you should take it seriously.

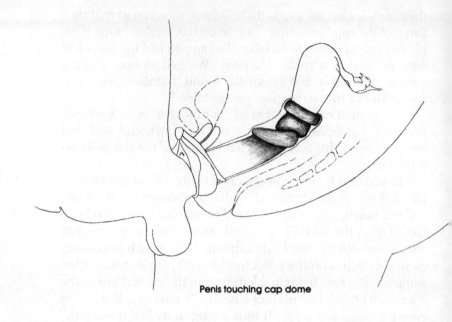

Penis touching cap dome

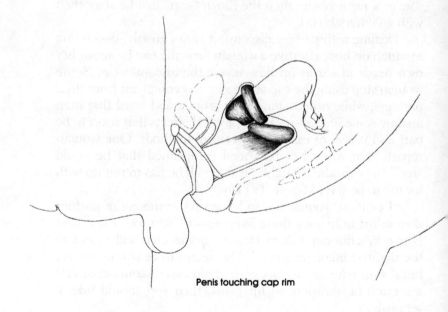

Penis touching cap rim

There is no way to tell ahead of time how the cap will feel to you or your partner, but 85 to 90 percent of men can't feel it, so it is reasonable to expect no problems.

DISLODGEMENT

The most perplexing problem for both cervical cap users and providers is the occasional unexplained dislodgement that many women experience at one time or another. Dislodgements also occur with the diaphragm, but much less often. Cervical cap investigators report that frequent dislodgements occur most often in the first few months of use, and that the frequency diminishes significantly with experience. Only 5 or 6 percent of cap users discontinue use for this reason.

Discovering the cap out of place can be very disconcerting, especially at first, but experienced users have been able to identify the cause of many displacements and take an occasional occurrence in stride. The most commonly mentioned causes of dislodgements are:

- Improper placement
- Poor fit
- Poor suction
- Vigorous intercourse or certain sexual positions
- Athletic activity
- Bowel movements
- Too much spermicide
- Heavy accumulation of cervical secretions or menstrual flow
- Severe fluid retention (edema)
- Cervix too close to vaginal opening or combination of short vagina and long penis
- Cervix entering the vagina at an angle
- Anteflexed or anteverted uterus

In instances where the dislodgement is noticed soon after intercourse, some practitioners suggest removing the cap and placing an applicator of spermicide in the vagina. However, it only takes about ninety seconds after ejaculation for sperm to get into the cervical canal and out of reach of all chemical weapons, so it isn't clear what good adding spermicide does, except to reassure yourself that you have done all you can do. If you discover that the cap is off the cervix when checking or removing it, try to determine the reason and watch for other incidents.

Note Because the cap is left in place longer and can be dislodged by activities other than intercourse, it needs to be checked more often. Until you are completely comfortable with your cap, *checking it faithfully before penetration and after intercourse and always using spermicide are your best defenses against dislodgement.*

You can encourage all of your sexual mates to be alert for dislodgements. "My boyfriend didn't tell me he noticed the dislodgement until the next morning," a Philadelphia woman says. "If he had mentioned that something felt unusual at the time, I would have asked him to ejaculate outside my vagina, or we could have gotten a condom."

"It doesn't happen very often, but the most clear-cut clue that my cap has slipped off is that either my partner or I will notice that spermicide has escaped into my vagina," a New York City attorney says.

It is often difficult to talk frankly about sexual activity, especially to male practitioners, but any details you can offer about sexual episodes during which a dislodgement occurs can be extremely helpful. Before your visit, you might review your situation: Was the sex particularly vigorous? Did you use a different or unusual position? Is your partner's penis especially large? How close is your cervix to the vaginal opening? Did you check your cap before and after intercourse? How much spermicide did you use? Did you have a strong bowel movement shortly before the dislodgement was discovered?

Repeated dislodgements may be indicative of a poor fit, so you may need a different size of cap. If your practitioner initially thought your fit was marginal, then a refit is definitely in order. You may be able to get a better fit the second time, as some women do, but if no better fit is obtained, you need to evaluate the risks of getting pregnant against continued cap use in light of your other options.

A few women appear to experience cap dislodgement with one partner and not another, while others find that they occur more frequently in certain sexual positions, such as rear entry or when the woman is on top. Cap users report occasional dislodgements associated with athletic activities or bowel movements. "I have found the cap can become dislodged in certain body positions when I do yoga, especially if my bowels are full," says one New York City medical researcher who uses the cap. However, many athletic women report no occurrences of dislodgement from vigorous activity and find the cap far more comfortable than the diaphragm.

Dr. Bernstein attempted to evaluate the role of fit in dislodgements, but was unable to come up with a definitive answer. "The rate of dislodgement does not appear to be directly related to the percent of subjects not fit or to the percent of subjects refit at a given clinic," he says. Nor does "the selectivity or experience of the fitting clinician . . . appear to offer a satisfactory explanation of the dislodgement rate." *

ODOR

Initially, the issue of odor buildup inside of the cervical cap received a great deal of attention because of Dr. Koch's report

---

* The impact of dislodgement on pregnancy rate has also been addressed by several other investigators. Dr. Neils Lauersen found a statistically significant correlation "between dislodgement at the time of intercourse and pregnancy, with 71 percent of thirty-nine women who became pregnant reporting cap displacement." Dr. Johan Eliot found that "cap dislodgement (reported by 31 percent of the study participants) . . . more than tripled the risk of pregnancy." And Dr. Koch has observed that "even a recipient whose Prentif cap meets all of the current fitting criteria faces some risk of dislodgement."

in *Contraception* * about the surprisingly high incidence of odor noticed by women in his study. After a good deal of medical sleuthing, he discovered that the oil-based Delfen cream, originally intended to be used alone as a vaginal spermicide, turned rancid inside the Prentif cap. After discovering this unique problem, Koch experimented with all of the commercial spermicidal preparations and eventually settled on the odorless, tasteless Ramses contraceptive cream. Many people prefer spermicides that are not medicinal tasting or perfumey, but any of the commercially available spermicidal creams or jellies (except foam) will work.† They all contain the same drug, nonoxynol-9, in similar amounts, so the differences are essentially cosmetic.

Unpleasant odor doesn't occur that frequently, but it can be a plague to some women, and its cause is often difficult to pin down. Over the years, both cap users and practitioners have discovered quite an array of home remedies that may eliminate or control odor:

• Reduce the period of wear.
• Alternate the use of two or three caps.
• Try soaking the cap for a few minutes in solutions of water and lemon juice, vinegar, baking soda, rubbing alcohol, bleach, or hydrogen peroxide.
• For vaginal odor, douche with povidone iodine (Betadine) and soak your cap in it. But nurse practitioner Jan Gerber, who fits caps in Duluth, Minnesota, has found the povidone iodine "eats" caps, so don't soak too long.
• Nurse practitioner Eileen Hatch recommends getting rid of vaginal/cap odor by inserting a gelatin capsule filled with powdered boric acid into the vagina.
• Peggy Norton, a nurse practitioner at the University of North Carolina Student Health Service, suggests cleaning the cap with fragrant oil of peppermint.

* James Koch, "The Prentif Cervical Cap: Acceptability Aspects and Their Implications for Future Design," *Contraception* 25(2), Feb. 1982.
† The bubbles from the aerosol foam may interfere with the suction of the Prentif by seeping under the rim.

• One Atlanta user says that she cleans her cap with toothpaste, with excellent results.

• A San Diego woman has two caps and cleans them with antibacterial soap.

• One woman who got her cap from the New Hampshire Feminist Health Center told her health worker that she had tried everything to deodorize the cap, and finally succeeded with coffee-pot cleaner.

• The Harvard Medical School Family Health Care Program suggests soaking odiferous caps in Cepacol.

• One frequently recommended home remedy is to add a few drops of liquid chlorophyll to the inside of the cap along with the spermicide.

If you have persistent odor problems, the best advice might be, "Try anything!"

Warning Cervical caps can "grow." Soaking overnight or longer may cause the rubber in the cap to expand and might eventually affect fit. If fifteen to thirty minutes isn't enough to get rid of odor, you probably ought to consult your practitioner to try to identify the cause and, perhaps, get a new cap.

THE CAUSES OF ODOR

Dr. Bernstein reports that in "the instances where malodor did develop, it was noticeable from both the cap and the diaphragm. He also found a definite "odor threshold" of three days or less for the cap. The women in Dr. Betty Schofield's Canadian study kept the cap in place for an average of fifty-three hours, and of those women who kept it in longer, some noted seventy-two hours as the odor threshold. The idea of an odor threshold has been mentioned by several other U.S. cap investigators. Some studies in which most participants tended to wear the cap for only one to two days at a time report almost no odor problems, indirectly corroborating the idea of an "odor threshold." On the other hand, Dr. Koch has found that many women in his study use the cap for longer periods without significant problems.

In efforts to discover the relationship between cap odor and vaginal bacteria, Dr. Bernstein and his colleagues conducted microbiological studies on ten women, culturing both the vagina and the inside of the caps after they had been worn for various lengths of time. Examinations of vaginal slides revealed that odor inside the caps was most frequently associated with the presence of *clue cells* which are indicative of *gardnerella vaginalis* (also called *hemophilus*). "Of the women with *clue cells*, 69 percent had malodor whereas only 20 percent of those without *clue cells* had this finding," the report says. "In another frame of reference, 75 percent of the women with cap malodor had *clue cells*, while 25 percent without odor had clue cells."

Independently, other practitioners have identified *gardnerella* as a primary cause of odor. In her practice in Cambridge, Massachusetts, nurse practitioner Mimi Secor has observed that odor is "more common in women who have undetected, asymptomatic *gardnerella* infections." Secor says that the odor usually disappears when the infection is treated. If you are having stubborn odor problems, it might be worthwhile to return to your practitioner for a vaginal culture, to see if you have an infestation of *gardnerella* or other bacteria in your vagina.

Note It is reassuring to know the cause of odor can usually be identified and treated.

The Bernstein report also found that odor could be caused by overgrowths of *bacteriodes* and/or *Proteus mirabilis*, two types of anaerobic bacteria normally found in the digestive tract that can cause an infectious reaction when they grow in large numbers in the vagina. The study also identified several other types of bacterial growths but did not find gonorrhea or chlamydia, the two major causes of pelvic inflammatory disease, suggesting that the cap plus nonoxynol-9 may offer protection against these more virulent pathogens.

A 1984 study conducted by the Ottawa Bureau of Medical Devices at the Department of National Health and Welfare in Canada investigated the problem of odor from a microscopic level. The authors collected nearly one hundred used Prentif caps and a few Vimules and examined them for discoloration, deterioration, and odors. Observing widespread signs of these conditions on the caps, which had been used from one month to three years, the authors concluded that the Prentif cap is "made of a particularly vulnerable rubber, with a tendency to become porous in contact with body fluids." Chemical analysis revealed "the presence of inorganic powders such as titanium oxides, chalks and other particulate 'fillers' . . . [used] to give opacity and flesh tones." The darker, heavier rubber of the few Vimules examined appeared to hold up better. The Atlanta Feminist Women's Health Center, which fit mostly Vimules when those caps were available in the United States, reports few odor problems from this period.

Dr. Lehfeldt, who has long been a champion of celluloid and lucite caps, says that there are virtually no odor problems with these materials no matter how long they are worn. Neither has odor developed as an issue with the silicon-based Contracap, which is intended to be left in place for up to one year. Perhaps the constitution of the rubber used in the Prentif—making this cap particularly vulnerable to the interactions with bacteria and bodily secretions—coupled with length of wear, is at the root of current odor problems.

In the future, odor that does not result from infections might be totally eliminated by the development of impermeable cap materials or of spermicides that also kill bacteria that cause odor.

BLEEDING

Women occasionally report noticing a trace of blood that is clearly not menstrual bleeding inside their caps upon removal. It seems to be fairly common for spotting to occur around the time of ovulation or during a routine speculum examination or Pap smear. Spotting during intercourse is probably quite common, but gets mixed in with semen and vaginal and cervical secretions and goes unnoticed. With the cap, any bleeding or spotting is prevented from mixing with vaginal secretions and is thus more noticeable.

Nurse Practitioner B. J. Bauermeister of the Blue Mountain Clinic in Missoula, Montana, suggests that bleeding of this nature can be disturbing to some women and that efforts should be made to reassure them that it is usually insignificant. Any unexplained bleeding that continues ought to be investigated, so if you discover blood inside of your cap frequently, note the amount and the time in your cycle that it occurs and mention it to your practitioner.

CERVICAL CHANGES

At the time of the reemergence of the cervical cap in the United States, some doctors expressed the fear that long-term use would cause adverse changes in the cervix, but this simply has not been the case. In order to evaluate the potential for cervical changes among cap users, Pap smears were done on all women entering cap studies and the issue was given special attention in the Bernstein study.

Throughout the six years of cap regulation, almost all of the cervical cap investigators reported that they have no more Pap smear conversions from Class I to Class II or III than in the general population. In Dr. Koch's study, where many women have been using the cap for five days or longer, very few changes have been noted. In his 1982 study Koch found that "observations of the effect of cap use on *erosions* . . . show rapid and healthy disappearance . . . with cap use in most cases and no change in the remaining cases." He also noted "14 conversions in a group of women using various methods of birth control and only 1 in the cap-wearing group, suggesting possible protective effects."

Unless there is some indication of a serious condition, Koch advises women of the possible risks and allows them to continue cap use. Many other practitioners, however, discourage women from using the cap in the presence of a Class II or Class III Pap smear reading, or postpone fitting a cap until the condition has been treated.

Bernstein and his colleagues found almost identical Pap smear conversion rates for both the cap and the diaphragm from Class I to Class II and from Class II to Class III, with rates for the cap being slightly lower in each case. Causes of conversions ranged from vaginitis and cervicitis to *gardnerella* and *papilloma* virus* and other cellular changes that are typical of all sexually active women. Bernstein did observe a higher rate of Pap smear conversions in cap users who were very sexually active. †

An abnormal Pap smear reading is one of the contraindications to cap use, but only until the condition has been resolved and the Pap smear reading has returned to Class I. Depending on the diagnosis, some women choose to use medication or home remedies, while others adopt a wait-and-see approach, since some conditions will clear up spontaneously. Common infections can cause the Pap smear reading to change from Class I to II or III, and the reading frequently returns to normal once the condition has been treated.

CONTRAINDICATIONS

Although the medical contraindications to cervical cap use are essentially the same as for the diaphragm, there are a few differences. If a woman cannot use the diaphragm because of repeated urinary-tract infections caused by pressure from the diaphragm rim on the urethra, she may be able to use the

---

* The human papilloma virus causes vaginal warts, and has been associated with pre-cancerous changes in some women.

† A higher rate of Pap smear changes occurs with all types of contraceptives in women who have multiple partners and are very sexually active and in women who are carriers of the potentially cancer-causing *papilloma* virus.

cervical cap without irritation. Women who have cystoceles or rectoceles (protrusions of the bladder or bowel through the vaginal wall) often have trouble using the diaphragm, but if the condition is not too severe, they may be able to use the cap successfully.

There seems to be general agreement that DES daughters and women who have a history of Toxic Shock Syndrome (TSS) should not use cervical caps, diaphragms or contraceptive sponges.

Note There have been several reports of the occurrence of Toxic Shock Syndrome with the diaphragm, but whether or not the diaphragm was the *direct cause* of the disease remains controversial. No cases of TSS have been reported with the cervical cap.

If you want to reduce the overall risk of TSS, do not use the cap, diaphragm or sponge during your menstrual period and remove it after six to eight hours. Do not use super-absorbent tampons and use tampons with inserters instead of the kind you insert with your fingers. Give your body a daily break from tampons by using a pad at night or switch to pads altogether. Also, be aware of the danger signs of TSS:

- A fever above 102°F.
- Vomiting
- Diarrhea
- Weakness or dizziness (from a sudden drop in blood pressure)
- Sunburn-like rash (often appears in later stages of the disease)

A survey of nearly one hundred cervical cap investigators yielded the following contraindications to cervical cap use:

• History of Toxic Shock Syndrome: Most practitioners agree that any woman who has had even a mild case of *diag-*

nosed TSS should not use the cap, diaphragm, or contraceptive sponge.

• DES daughter: DES daughters are in a particularly difficult situation regarding birth control. There is almost nothing that is thought to be non-irritating to the cervix in some way. However, most practitioners are in agreement that a woman who has already been exposed to DES should not use a device that fits right over the cervix, since this might exacerbate an already volatile condition.

• History of or current pelvic inflammatory disease (PID): Most practitioners will fit a cap after you have been symptom-free for one year.

• Unresolved abnormal Pap smear: Many Class II Pap smear readings are the result of infection or irritation and are not "pre-cancerous" conditions. Often treatment will alleviate the irritation and a cap can then be fitted.

• Allergy to spermicide or rubber: If the allergy is mild and reaction is not too severe, you (or your partner) may decide to seek treatment, but if the reaction is severe, treatments may not be effective. Some women with allergies to spermicide use their caps without it.

• Poor fit: This is one of the most controversial contraindications to cap use. Since the percentage of women fit varies from practitioner to practitioner, if you are told that you have a poor fit, a second opinion would definitely be worthwhile.

• Very long or very short cervix: On a long cervix, the cap rim is not protected by the vaginal musculature and may be more vulnerable to dislodgement; if the neck of the cervix is very short, the cap will simply not have enough to hold on to. A cervix that enters the vagina at an angle may leave part of the cap rim exposed.

• Discomfort with touching genitals: Because of social conditioning, some women are truly squeamish or timid about touching their genitals and need special encouragement and support.

• Difficulty with insertion or removal: Although a small percentage of women may experience seemingly insurmountable difficulties at first, time, patience, motivation, and above all *practice* can solve most problems associated with insertion or removal.

• Current vaginal infection: These include chlamydia, condyloma (vaginal warts), trichomoniasis, *gardnerella* (homophilus), *actinomyces israelii* or nonspecific vaginitis. Once these conditions are cleared up, you can begin or resume cap use.

• Asymmetrical cervix or obstetrical damage: Deep lacerations from childbirth may leave the cervix too irregular to accommodate the fairly rigid rim of the Prentif cap.

• Prolapsed uterus (cervix close to vaginal opening): If the cervix is too close to the vaginal opening, the cap may be more susceptible to dislodgement or cause user or partner discomfort. Some surgical remedies are available for this condition, if you are highly motivated to use the cap.

• Nabothian cysts: While these cysts are considered harmless, a large one near where the rim of the cap grips the cervix may interfere with suction or fit. The rim may also irritate the cyst. Removal of the cyst may need to be done before cap use is undertaken.

Because women have so few birth control options, cap practitioners have generally taken a very liberal approach to contraindications, working with highly motivated women to help them overcome many conditions so that they can use the cap safely. Dr. Gary Richwald and his colleagues in the Los Angeles Cervical Cap Study found that about 40 percent of women who asked for a cap but were initially rejected could be fit once their conditions improved.

The high satisfaction rates reported in almost every cervical cap study suggest that problems occur for small percentages of women and that when they do, they can often be effectively worked through.

8 ✳ SEX AND SPONTANEITY:
Good News from Couples
and Researchers

In instances where the diaphragm does interfere with sensation, one answer may be the use of the cervical cap.
—Alice Kahn Ladas, Beverly Whipple,
and John Perry
The G Spot

Barrier methods have a reputation, which may or may not be deserved, for putting a damper on sexual spontaneity and interfering, in one way or another, with erogenous feeling. Women and their partners often adjust to the small inconveniences of barrier methods and use them very effectively, but admit to secretly hoping for something a little less intrusive. They may not have dreamed in vain. Many women have praised the cap's convenience and the freedom from the demands of daily insertion and removal, reporting a marked improvement in both their desire for sex and a significant increase in the frequency of intercourse. These experiences have been documented by the most prominent cervical cap investigators as well as by some well-known sex researchers who have directly addressed the cap's positive impact on sexuality.

In 1982, Dr. James Koch reported that 19 percent of the respondents to a questionnaire acknowledged an increase in sex drive and 29 percent noted an increase in the frequency of intercourse. Dr. Bernstein also noted that in his study "more cap users than diaphragm users reported that their device did not interfere with sex . . . and a higher percentage of the cap users continue to comment on . . . increased spontaneity associated with cap use."

Although many people have perfectly satisfactory, even outstanding, sex with the diaphragm, others object to the messiness, the medicinal or perfumey taste of spermicides, and what some refer to as the "rubber raincoat effect" of having half of the vagina covered by the device's latex dome.

The spongy tissue running along the roof of the vagina and surrounding the urethra has recently been the subject of some interest to sex researchers. This structure, similar to that which surrounds the male urethra in the penis, has been identified by a sexuality study project of the Federation of Feminist Women's Health Centers and named the "urethral sponge." It has also been designated by researchers Alice Ladas, Beverly Whipple, and John Perry as the location of the so-called G spot.* Even though the urethral sponge can be touched either by fingers or by the penis during sexual activity with the diaphragm in place, for many people there is no substitute for the sensation of skin-to-skin contact. Although the rubber used in diaphragms is quite thin, its slick rubber surface can cut down on friction, which is extremely pleasurable to both men and women, and inhibits exploration of this very sensitive area with fingers.

The issue of the diaphragm's interference with women's sexual sensation is not new. As early as 1944, two extremely influential sex researchers—Dr. Ernest Grafenberg, for whom the "G spot" is named, and Dr. Robert Latou Dickinson— noted, "Occasionally, a patient has reported failure to reach orgasm wearing a vaginal diaphragm. . . . Because the cervix cap leaves the interior wall uncovered, whereas the diaphragm covers it, these patients can obtain orgasm after the change is

---

* According to Ladas, Whipple, and Perry, the G spot is located on "a complex network of blood vessels, the paraurethral glands and ducts, nerve endings and tissue surrounding the bladder neck." They have suggested that this spot may be more intensely sensitive in some women. They say, however, that not all women have a "G spot" and that its exact location can differ from woman to woman. The Feminist Women's Health Centers study found the idea of a "spot" too limiting, suggesting instead that all women have a urethral sponge, that it becomes erect during sexual response, and that it is highly sensitive to the touch. They emphasize, however, that *it is not necessary to touch the urethral sponge to have an orgasm.* See The Federation of Feminist Women's Health Centers, *A New View of a Woman's Body* (New York: Simon & Schuster, 1982), and Alice Kahn Ladas, Beverly Whipple, and John Perry, *The G Spot and Other Recent Discoveries in Human Sexuality* (New York: Henry Holt & Co., 1982).

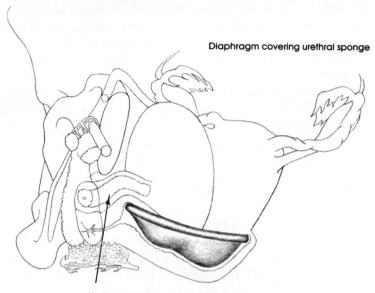

Diaphragm covering urethral sponge

Urethral sponge

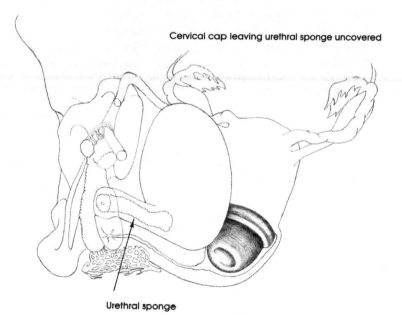

Cervical cap leaving urethral sponge uncovered

Urethral sponge

made."* As noted above, it is not necessary to touch the urethral sponge with either the fingers or the penis to achieve orgasm, but stimulation of this structure, which is less effective through the diaphragm dome, may be very desirable for some women.

There has been some suggestion, as yet undocumented except by occasional anecdotal reports, that the cap's tight grip on the cervix may enhance uterine contractions for certain women during sexual response. Barbara Seaman noted this phenomenon in *Women and the Crisis in Sex Hormones*, reporting the experience of a friend who firmly believed that her cap "enhanced intercourse." This is certainly an intriguing concept that deserves future investigation.

Some men don't like being able to feel the cap, but others say that touching the cap with the penis is pleasurable and actually enhances sensation. "I found that rubbing the tip of the glans against the cap rim heightened sensation enormously," says an artist from San Diego.

A few men also report that they are turned on by helping their partners insert the cap before penetration occurs. "I always felt a little left out where birth control was concerned," admits an accountant from Seattle. "But now when my girlfriend lets me insert her cap, it makes me feel really good and I think I try a little harder to please her."

For a few couples, the cap can be uncomfortable and may have a negative effect on sex. Once in a while a woman can experience discomfort from the cap, especially if she has a short vagina and her partner has a long penis. More often, the penis may hit the firm edge of the Prentif too hard and the man can experience discomfort as well.

One of the diaphragm's well-known foibles is the tendency for the spermicide to ooze out of the vagina onto the clitoral lips, causing both women and men to complain that oral sex is less enjoyable, or downright distasteful.† With the cervical cap, there may be a little residue of spermicide on the lips if

* Ernest Grafenberg and Robert L. Dickinson, "Conception Control by Plastic Cervical Cap," *Western Journal of Surgery, Obstetrics & Gynecology* 52(8), Aug. 1944, pp. 336–37.

† See page 121 for a warning on oral sex and AIDS.

	CERV. CAP	DIA-PHRAGM	SPONGE	PILL	IUD	CON-DOM	SPERMI-CIDES	NAT. FAM. PLAN-NING	OUTER-COURSE	FEMALE STERIL.	VASEC-TOMY	ABOR-TION	WITH-DRAWAL
Must be used for each act of intercourse to be effective	yes	yes	yes	yes	yes	yes	yes	no	yes	n/a	n/a	no	yes
Can interfere with spontaneity	maybe	maybe	maybe	no	no	yes	yes	yes	no	no	no	no	maybe
Must be used during periods of sexual inactivity	no	no	no	yes	yes	no	no	no	no	yes	yes	no	no
Effect on libido	may inc.	may dec.	may dec.	may dec.	none	may dec.	may dec.	none	none	none	none	none	none
Effect on vaginal lubrication	none	may inc.	may dec.	may dec.	none	none	may inc.	none	none	none	none	none	none
Protects against sexually transmissible diseases	some	yes	some	no*	no	yes†	yes	no	yes	none	some	none	some
Requires good communication	no	no	no	no	no	yes	yes	yes	yes	no	no	no	yes
Promotes better communication and sexual expression	maybe	maybe	maybe	no	no	maybe	maybe	yes	yes	no	no	no	no
Can be messy	no	yes	no	no	no	no	yes	no	no	no	no	no	no
Responsibility	♀	♀	♀	♀	♀	♀♂	♀♂	♀♂	♀♂	♀	♂	♀	♂

*The Pill protects against more severe forms of pelvic inflammatory disease, but not against those caused by chlamydia.

† The condom is the only birth-control method that offers protection against the AIDS virus. Nonoxynol-9, the sperm-killing ingredient in spermicides approved in the United States, has been found to kill the virus in a test tube, but further studies are necessary before its effectiveness is fully known.

you put the cap in just before sex, but it can be easily wiped away with a damp washcloth.

The Pill is generally considered to be the ideal method of birth control as far as sex is concerned, but it too has its drawbacks. Some women experience a definite decrease in libido, sometimes for lengthy periods, and may not even recognize it until several months after discontinuing the Pill. Others suffer from vaginal dryness, caused by the suppression in estrogen production, especially from combined Pills. If you are a Pill user and think your desire for sex is less than it was before you started the Pill, you might consider switching to the cap for a while and see if your sex drive improves. For anyone experiencing vaginal dryness, the diaphragm is probably ideal, because the spermicide acts as a vaginal lubricant and more can always be added as needed.

THE IMPACT OF BIRTH CONTROL ON SEXUALITY

The following chart is designed to help you see at a glance how the available methods of birth control compare in terms of their effects on sexuality. Of course, no method is ideal. When comparing them, however, it is important to remember that sex is highly individual and that these categories are only generalizations, representing the way many, but not all, people experience certain sexual phenomena.

9 ✳ YOUNG WOMEN AND THE CAP:
A New Option to Consider Seriously

As punks have eagerly adopted the fashion of piercing their
ears numerous times, and even their nasal septa, they could
also decide for cervical jewelry, individually cast gold and
silver or plastic caps, to be worn as ornaments when not in
situ, perhaps. Women less eager to épater the squeamish
might like to pretend that it is some piece of zoomorphic
artwork (which it is) and keep the secret of its function to
themselves.

—Germaine Greer
Sex and Destiny

One of the most impenetrable tenets in the family-planning
canon is that adolescents, and even young women of college
age, cannot and will not use barrier methods effectively. Yet
this pervasive orthodoxy is based almost entirely on "custom
and usage" rather than upon verifiable scientific data and remains open to discussion.

The situation young people find themselves in today regarding sexuality and birth control is appalling. Teenagers are
more sexually active than ever before, but their level of realistic, concrete information about sex and reproduction is woe-
fully inadequate, and the major contraceptive method used
by adults—surgical sterilization—is singularly inappropriate
for them. The Pill, used by 40 percent of young women, is
also inappropriate for certain substantial subgroups such as
those who smoke, heavy alcohol or drug users, those whose
hormonal cycles are not yet fully established, and the considerable number of young Pill users who discontinue use because of unwanted physical effects. Citing health problems
and the irregularity of sexual activity among many adolescents, Judith Bruce and S. Bruce Schearer of the Population

Council argue that "continuous use of oral contraceptives or an IUD among [teenagers] can be seen as overmedication that exposes users not only to the inherent risks of these methods, but also to additional unnecessary risks because the method is being used for long periods with no purpose."*

RECONSIDERING BARRIER METHODS

Scant research exists on barrier methods in general, and almost none on their use by teenagers. Nevertheless, it seems essential that we examine with open minds the basis of the assumption that these methods are irrelevant to young people at the time when a new and better barrier method, the cervical cap, is becoming generally available.

The case for reconsideration of the use of the cervical cap, diaphragm, and other barrier methods by young people has been made by some of the most highly placed and influential researchers in the field of contraception. Referring to a study directed by Dr. Mary Lane at the Margaret Sanger Research Bureau in New York City in 1976,† Dr. Robert Hatcher and the staff of *Contraceptive Technology* assert that "very effective use [of the diaphragm] has been documented for young nulliparous women and teenagers, so age should not be accepted as a valid reason to discourage diaphragm use." This study found a 98 percent effectiveness rate and 80 percent continuation at the end of one year for women under 18 years of age.

Bruce and Schearer note that "large providers in different parts of the country have begun to prescribe diaphragms for as many as one fifth of their teenage clients. Recent studies show that with adequate instruction and support, these young users are obtaining very high effectiveness." Dr. Mary Calde-

* Judith Bruce and S. Bruce Schearer, *Contraception and Common Sense* (The Population Council, 1 Dag Hammerskjold Plaza, New York, 1979), p. 41
† Mary Lane, R. Arleo, and A.J. Sobrero, "Successful Use of the Diaphragm and Jelly in a Young Population: Report of a Clinical Study," *Family Planning Perspectives*, vol. 2, no. 2, pp. 81–86.

rone, whose 1972 textbook* included an in-depth chapter on the cervical cap by Dr. Lehfeldt, believes that the cap is "probably far more appropriate and safe than the Pill, provided that a girl can learn to place it."

Ruth Bell, a member of the Boston Women's Health Book Collective and the author of *Changing Bodies, Changing Lives*, a health book for teenagers, observed positive reaction to the cervical cap during a tour of birth control clinics for young people across the United States. "Many girls and women are enthusiastic about the cervical cap because . . . it will be the first birth control device that is effective and free from dangerous side effects *that doesn't have to be applied each time before intercourse.*" †

OBSTACLES IN THE PROVISION OF BARRIER METHODS

In analyzing problems in the provision of barrier methods to adolescents and young adults, both *Contraceptive Technology* and the Population Council identify practitioner bias as one of the primary stumbling blocks. A poll of family-planning practitioners conducted by *Contraceptive Technology* documents a clear-cut and almost aggressive bias against the diaphragm and other barriers, and an active preference for the Pill. "Service providers exert a major influence on the acceptability of barrier contraceptives," the Population Council notes. "Simply put, motivation and knowledge being equal, a person who visits a clinic that supports barrier methods is more likely to use them." The report also notes, "Some members of the medical community have apprehensions about the increasing reliance of adolescents on the Pill and IUD. This apprehension, however, has not yet been translated into enthusiasm for barrier methods."

Confirming teenagers' susceptibility to practitioner bias,

* Mary S. Calderone, *Manual of Family Planning and Contraceptive Practice* (Baltimore: The Williams & Wilkins Co., 1979).

† Ruth Bell, *Changing Bodies, Changing Lives* (New York: Random House, 1980).

Family Planning Perspectives points out, "Teenage clients not only expect and want the clinician to tell them what method they should get, but they are more likely to be consistent users of an effective method when they attend clinics where such guidance is given. . . . The highest and most significant positive correlation [of a study of almost three thousand teenagers] was with the adolescents' desire to have the nurses tell them what contraceptive to use." *

An outgrowth of practitioners' bias toward the Pill is that young people suffer from a severe lack of information about the safety, effectiveness, and positive benefits of barrier methods, as well as information about how they work and how to circumvent or minimize their inconveniences.

Changing Bodies, Changing Lives, an account by a sixteen-year-old Los Angeles high school student, provides an illustration of how a supportive clinic atmosphere can easily demystify barrier methods for young women and, at the same time, give them much-needed positive information about their bodies:

> I used to think I'd never be able to use a diaphragm because it was creepy for me to even think about putting it in. I thought that whole area down there was sort of disgusting. But one day [at] the women's clinic near our school . . . they did this demonstration for us, where they showed us their cervix . . . and some of the girls in the class even did it. . . . It was really amazing. Everybody's cervix looked a little different. Some were big, some were little, some holes were open pretty big and some were pretty tight. Then they showed us how the diaphragm goes in and covers up that hole. It made it seem logical.

As this illustration suggests, a lack of information is a major factor in young women's disinterest in barrier methods.

* *Family Planning Perspectives* 17 (5), Sept./Oct. 1985, p. 223.

THE TREND AWAY FROM THE PILL

In spite of the aggressive marketing of the Pill to young people, its use among adolescents decreased in the late 1970s, following the trend in the general population. The movement away from high-risk methods, and increased reliance on condoms and withdrawal by young people, reflects a genuine concern about both health and fertility risks and makes an even stronger argument for the promotion of effective barrier methods.

"Slowly it is being recognized that adolescents are a heterogeneous group and that they will—and should—seek individual solutions compatible with their personal habits, preferences and concerns for safety and effectiveness," the Population Council report concludes.

THE CERVICAL CAP AND YOUNG WOMEN

If there is a trend away from the Pill toward more low-risk methods among teenagers, then there is a strong argument to be made for the promotion of the cervical cap as a contraceptive option.

While obtaining a cap requires a visit to a clinic or physician and must be inserted and removed manually, it has the advantage of not being as awkward and messy as the diaphragm can be. Its use can be separated from sex and it offers protection against many sexually transmitted diseases. The cervical cap fitting also offers an excellent opportunity for young women to become acquainted with their reproductive anatomy in a supportive environment.

It is significant that upon FDA approval, the cap will be provided by all Planned Parenthood clinics. No doubt the support of this influential organization will have an impact on state and locally funded family-planning clinics, which are heavily utilized by teenagers. If practitioners in this nationwide network of clinics are positive and enthusiastic about the cervical cap, it could serve as a viable alternative for many young women who need birth control, but who cannot or do not want to take the Pill.

10 ✳ EFFECTIVENESS RATES:
Results of the FDA Cap Studies

In the long-awaited FDA-mandated study comparing the Prentif cavity rim cervical cap and the diaphragm, the two devices yielded almost identical effectiveness rates for typical users: 82.6 percent for the cap and 83.3 percent for the diaphragm. For perfect users, women who used their caps for every session of intercourse, the cap was 93.6 percent effective. Many other studies conducted concurrently under FDA guidelines, listed on the chart on pages 192–196, found effectiveness rates ranging from the high 80s to the high 90s. What do these variations in statistics mean? Just how effective is the cervical cap? In order to answer these questions accurately, we need some basic information on how to interpret birth control statistics.

USE EFFECTIVENESS VERSUS THEORETICAL EFFECTIVENESS

The Pill is 99 percent effective, right? Not exactly. The Pill is effective approximately 99.5 percent of the time for an ideal woman who has an ideal life with no major health problems, who never forgets to take her Pill, and who has sex no more than three times a week. That's called *theoretical effectiveness*. There is another effectiveness rate, called *use effectiveness*, which describes the chances of getting pregnant for the woman whose prescription runs out over a holiday weekend, the one who gets sick and doesn't take her Pills, the one who loses her packet on a two-week camping trip in the High Sierras, or the one who frequently forgets to take them for any number of reasons. For these women, use effectiveness can drop as low as 96 percent. Further, the use effectiveness of the mini-pill is less than that of the stronger *combined* oral contraceptives. For Pills, there is yet another use-effectiveness rate: 94.5 percent for teenagers, who tend to take Pills more erratically than older, more mature women. The use effectiveness of any method differs from study to study, depending upon a host of factors, all of which must be taken into account when evaluating birth control statistics.

Note Birth control statistics are now frequently given in terms of *failure rates*, but because women typically want to know "how effective" a method is, the data in this handbook will be rendered in terms of *effectiveness* rather than in terms of *failure* even though the translation is not exact. For example, if the Pill has a 4 percent failure rate, it can be said to have a 96 percent effectiveness rate.

All of the effectiveness rates for the Pill are within about five or six percentage points of each other. The case of the diaphragm is far more complicated. The theoretical-effectiveness rate—when it is used consistently and correctly for every single incidence of intercourse, again, by an ideal woman with an ideal life—is about 98 percent, as good as that of the Pill. But use-effectiveness rates for the diaphragm range anywhere from a high of 98.1 percent to the low 80s. And no wonder. The way in which women use the diaphragm varies widely. Some use the diaphragm every time they have intercourse, and some only use it about two weeks each cycle when they think they may be fertile. Some add spermicide for every session of intercourse, and some don't. Some find themselves without it on an unexpected encounter, and some leave it in the drawer on a cold night.

Such variations in usage can produce widely differing use-effectiveness rates for the various methods. A recent example of such differences arose in comparing the diaphragm to both the cap and the contraceptive sponge. In the FDA study conducted by Dr. Bernstein, the diaphragm produced an 83 percent effectiveness rate when compared to the cervical cap, but it was found to be 87 percent effective in a comparative study with the Today™ contraceptive sponge.* While this discrepancy is major, it is considered perfectly acceptable within current research standards and would be attributed to variations in study population, usage, and standards set by individual researchers.

One way to look at use effectiveness is to distinguish between the *highest observed effectiveness rate* (the highest use-effectiveness rate found in any single study) and the *typical-user effectiveness* rate (an average of the results of several studies evaluating use effectiveness). For example, the authors of *Contraceptive Technology*, who have done extensive comparative analyses of birth control statistics, found the highest observed effectiveness rate for the diaphragm to be 98.1 percent in a study conducted by Dr. Mary Lane, but found the typical-user effectiveness rate to be 81 percent, an average derived from a number of studies. Apparently, the women in Dr. Lane's study used the diaphragm correctly and faithfully, and their use-effectiveness rate approached the device's theoretical effectiveness.

Dr. Bernstein likes to compare the difference in theoretical-effectiveness and use-effectiveness rates to mileage estimates for cars. A finely tuned new car with an expert driver and ideal driving conditions might get thirty-five miles per gallon. However, the average four-year-old car (same make, same model, same gas) that is driven from home to school to the supermarket and then to the beach in heavy traffic will get fewer miles per gallon. And a car that is out of tune, has worn-out tires, and runs on cheap gas will do even worse.

---

* S. L. McIntyre and J. E. Higgins, "Factors Related to Pregnancy Rates Obtained by Contraceptive Sponge Users" (Paper presented to the Association for Planned Parenthood Professionals, Nov. 2–3 1984).

LIFE TABLE ANALYSIS VERSUS PEARL INDEX

Another important factor in evaluating birth control studies is knowing whether the statistics were computed according to the Life Table Analysis method or the Pearl Index, a statistical method now considered outdated by some. The *Pearl Index* gives an effectiveness or failure rate "per 100 woman-years of exposure" to intercourse. The flaw in this way of looking at effectiveness rates is that the method is open-ended. The longer a study runs, and the more woman-years it tallies, the better the rate will be. Experienced women use a method more effectively over time, while less motivated ones drop out, resulting in higher effectiveness rates.

Life Table Analysis poses this question: "Out of one hundred women using a particular method, how many will become pregnant in one year?" The answer might be "four out of a hundred," which can also be rendered in terms of effectiveness as "96 percent of one hundred women." This way of looking at effectiveness supposedly shows a more accurate typical-user effectiveness rate than the Pearl Index.

THE EFFECT OF STUDY POPULATION ON EFFECTIVENESS RATES

In designing a study, researchers keep a careful eye on a host of factors that can affect, in some cases dramatically, the study outcome. Cultural, religious, and economic values and motivations regarding pregnancy can alter the outcome of two otherwise identically designed studies. Dr. Bernstein contends rather cynically that "you can get any result you want if you design your study right.* For example, a study of diaphragm use in Italy, where the Catholic Church has an aggressive

---

* This is decidedly an unsettling notion, but has been shown to be true over and over. It remains to other researchers and consumer advocates to critique important studies of contraceptive use to alert women and the media to unethical practices in research and analysis. Barbara Seaman did just that in 1981 when she spoke out across the country against the Walnut Creek study of the Pill, which was so flawed that even the U.S. government withdrew its funding.

anti–birth control stance, might be far different than one conducted in Sweden, which has a strong sex-education program in public schools and very supportive social and official attitudes toward the use of contraceptives. The outcome of a study on married couples in Japan, where the condom is the major method of birth control, might be far different from one on condom use by teenagers in the United States, who are known to be erratic users of contraceptives.

The basic fertility of the study population is an important consideration and can be very influential on effectiveness rates. For example, a group of prostitutes who have had high exposure to sexually transmitted diseases might have a high degree of infertility, and thus achieve higher effectiveness rates than a group of women who have been monogamous for long periods of time.

Women who have frequent intercourse, say five or six times a week, will have lower effectiveness rates than women who have sex less often, say once or twice a week. And whether many women in a particular study consider that they have finished their childbearing or plan to have more children can also affect study outcome.

The issue of "risk taking" in contraceptive effectiveness rates is a significant one. Effectiveness rates for all methods tend to be higher for women who say they do not want any more children, and rates are generally higher for women who have never been pregnant—and perhaps take fewer risks—than for those who have. In the specific instance of the cervical cap, the Bernstein study showed a lower effectiveness rate for women who said that they initiated sexual activity before the age of sixteen, suggesting that early sexual activity may be indicative of risk-taking in terms of birth control.

USER FAILURES VERSUS METHOD FAILURES

Effectiveness rates are often looked at in terms of *user failures* or *method failures*. For surgical sterilization and IUDs, the user failure is roughly the same, since there is very little chance for human error. But in the case of the diaphragm or the cervical cap, where patterns of use can vary, rates differ significantly. Leaving the diaphragm in the drawer and getting pregnant is a *user failure*. Using it every time, but getting pregnant anyway, is a *method failure*. In comparing the cervical cap and the diaphragm, Dr. Bernstein found that the diaphragm had a slightly lower rate of user effectiveness at one year (87.4 percent compared to 88.3 percent) while the cervical cap had a lower rate of method effectiveness for the same period (93.6 percent compared to 96.4 percent). Women in this particular study appeared to use the cap more faithfully than the diaphragm, but the cap itself failed slightly more often. Yet the effectiveness rate was virtually the same.

Some analysts have suggested that use-effectiveness statistics for various methods might be lower if it were possible to include data for women who discontinue a method for medical reasons, because of unwanted physical effects, or because they disliked the method and got pregnant before choosing another method. Thus far, no one has researched this intriguing, and possibly significant, question.

FOLLOW-UP

The intensity with which follow-up is pursued and the manner in which it is done is a critical factor that can strongly affect study outcome. In the case of the cervical cap, some investigators required follow-up visits, while others did most follow-up by way of a questionnaire. Some had high follow-up rates, while others—which served more transient populations such as college students or included many women who drove long distances to get caps—lost many study participants, and possibly many pregnancies, to follow-up.

These distinctions are especially important in regard to the cervical cap because many of the studies which were conducted in concurrence with the Bernstein study had different goals, standards, methodologies, and study populations, and their results, looked at together, can be confusing to the lay person.

What does all this mean about the cap's effectiveness? It means that there is no one single effectiveness rate that is more valid than others, that each study is valid for its own study population, study design and implementation. Any birth control method with as much possibility for variation in use, such as the cervical cap or the diaphragm, is bound to have a wide range of effectiveness rates. In that case perhaps it is best to look at the typical-user effectiveness rate as one generalization, rather than at the theoretical or highest observed effectiveness rate, keeping in mind, though, that careful and consistent use of the cap may approach the latter two categories in effectiveness. If women know how to use a method effectively, they will probably use it better. Good users in every study will have fewer pregnancies than inconsistent users.

THE BERNSTEIN REPORT

Dr. Bernstein found 17.4 cap failures per hundred women for one year. This figure includes both user failures and method failures, and translates into a typical-user effectiveness rate of 82.6 percent. For women who did not use their caps for every session of intercourse, there were 11.7 failures for every hundred women, or an 88.3 percent effectiveness rate. For women who said that they used their caps correctly for every session of intercourse there were 6.4 failures per hundred women, yielding an effectiveness rate of 93.6 percent, *more than 10 percent better than for inconsistent users*. These two figures combined equal a typical-user effectiveness rate of 82.6 percent. The figures for perfect use clearly show that the cervical cap can be extremely effective—almost as effective as the IUD.

The report also computed separate effectiveness-rate analyses which show how the cap works for certain subgroups of women. For example, cap effectiveness for college graduates was 89.4 percent, but 73.1 percent for women with only a high-school education or less. Unmarried cap users appeared to use the cap far more effectively than married users, 84.2 percent for unmarried users compared to 73.2 percent for those who were married. (This was an expected outcome based on the results of many other studies comparing contraceptive use in married and unmarried users. Married people seem to take more risks, possibly because a failure may be more acceptable, at least theoretically, than to single women.) The rates between older and younger women did not differ significantly, but women with prior diaphragm experience had an 88.7 percent effectiveness rate, while women who had never used a diaphragm had an 82 percent effectiveness rate. Women who had never had an abortion had an effectiveness rate of 86.6 percent, while women who had a history of at least one previous abortion had only a 79 percent effectiveness rate. Finally, women who were extremely sexually active had considerably lower effectiveness rates—75.5 percent for women who had sex more than three times a week—while women who had intercourse one to three times a week had a higher rate, 85.4 percent. Women who had sex less than once a week had an effectiveness rate of 88.9 percent.

These statistics suggest the profile of the *ideal* cervical cap user: an unmarried college graduate who initiated sexual activity after the age of sixteen, has previous diaphragm experience, has never been pregnant, and does not have sex more than about once a week. *But this is only a statistical profile* and does not take into account other very influential factors in effective cap use such as user motivation, consistent use, confidence, partner cooperation, future intentions about pregnancy, and perhaps the "desperation factor." There is no doubt that in every study, many successful users can be found who do not fit this statistical stereotype.

The Bernstein report is useful in certain significant respects, but also has some outstanding deficiencies. Perhaps the most obvious is that it tells us little about the range of experience women have with the cap. None of the study participants wore the cap for more than three days, and none of them had the option to not use spermicide. Both of the sperm transport studies (noted earlier in this chapter) and the microbiology study (discussed in conjunction with odor problems on page 84) were done on so few women as to be inconclusive, and they were not done on diaphragm users for comparative purposes. Although this study identified certain problems with the cap, it completely fails to address the critical issue of solutions. The all-important question of fit was addressed only cursorily, although eight study sights, some of them serviced by the same practitioner, offered an ideal opportunity to investigate some of the anomalies in fitting criteria. Throughout the study, each woman kept a detailed diary of her day-by-day experiences with the cap. This mountain of data must include illuminating information about all aspects of cap use—how women like the cap, what they see as its drawbacks, how their partners feel about it, and the cap's effect on sexuality—yet there is almost no reference to this material in the report except in statistical form. Perhaps some of this valuable information will be forthcoming in future reports by Dr. Bernstein and his colleagues in medical journals.

OTHER CAP STUDIES

Concurrent with the Bernstein study, the FDA allowed nearly one hundred individual practitioners and clinics to dispense caps under Investigational Device Exemptions (IDEs), with the stipulation that each IDE holder collect follow-up data and submit it to the agency on an annual basis. The requirements established for applying for an IDE were relatively uncomplicated, and FDA officials aided prospective investigators in setting up acceptable study designs. Yet, in establishing these guidelines the agency asked for certain data, but failed to specify any particular format or method of analysis, making comparisons and analysis of the studies difficult if not impossible. Even though the FDA required investigators to attempt to follow each woman by questionnaire and submit an annual report, it has steadfastly maintained that it has no intention of evaluating the data or publishing the information in any form. Almost all of the IDE holders have criticized this decision, complaining that they were required to follow elaborate and expensive data collection procedures only to have their painstaking reports end up in the FDA dustbin.

The chart on pages 191–195 contains data from nearly one hundred IDE holders who actively provided caps during the five-year study period. A few of these studies (noted with an * and listed in the Bibliography) have been published, but most of them have not. The reports from which this data was extracted contain not only statistics on effectiveness, but invaluable information about day-to-day cervical cap use which appears through this book, dispelling myths about cap use and documenting real-life solutions to problems. The reports are fascinating in both the similarities they disclose and the differences in experience they reveal.

Because of the varied and sometimes eccentric formats of these reports, it is difficult to draw hard conclusions, but some illuminating general trends can be seen. For example, almost all of the effectiveness rates, especially those arrived at by Life Table Analysis, are higher than those reported by Bernstein, with many in the 88 to 95 percent range. In spite of considerable disagreement over fit, many practitioners fit from 75 to 85 percent of the women who ask for caps, while a few fit higher percentages. Although the issue of spermicide use with the Prentif is yet to be resolved, these studies show that some women are eschewing its use, at least part of the time. The investigators exhibit an overwhelming preference for the size 22 Prentif, followed by size 25, although it is apparent that a few practitioners fit larger, and have similar effectiveness rates. Finally, the studies show a definite conservative trend in cap wear of one to three days, but also reveal quite a bit of variation in length of wear.

An overwhelming majority of women in the cap studies were white, college educated, and middle class. In addition, as Lehfeldt and Sivin point out in their study, the population of women who sought the cap during the FDA study period were highly self-selected. Implied in this observation is the probability that many of the study participants were more highly motivated to use their method correctly. Ruth Polotta, cap study administrator at the Elizabeth Blackwell Clinic for Women in Philadelphia, points out another outstanding characteristic of women who sought out the cap. "I call it the 'desperation factor,'" she says. "Many of the women who come in for the cap have *tried everything* and had bad results. They will do anything to make it work."

Another significant aspect of these cervical cap studies is that with the exception of Dr. Bernstein's, which was funded by NICHHD, all of the studies were conducted by very committed pro–cervical cap practitioners. As a result, there is no doubt some element of pro–cap practitioner bias in the design and implementation of these studies. However, without their foresight and acute awareness of the need for new, low-risk contraceptive options, the cap would have been completely unavailable throughout the long FDA study period.

11 ✳ COMPARISON SHOPPING:
A Comprehensive Survey of
Birth Control Options

"After getting phlebitis on the Pill, getting pregnant with the diaphragm, and being scared by a difficult IUD removal, I was ecstatic to hear about the reborn cervical cap," a twenty-eight-year-old Washington, D.C., woman says.*

"I stopped using the Pill because I smoke," another Washington, D.C., resident recalls. "And I had my IUD removed before an extended trip overseas in case any complications developed. Then I was told by several doctors I could not use a diaphragm because of a retroverted uterus. In the meantime, I got pregnant twice."*

There are no exact figures, but birth control practitioners report that they see women every day whose contraceptive experience is similar to that described by the two women above.

With the abrupt withdrawal of IUDs from the U.S. market in 1985 and 1986, the media finally came to recognize what women and researchers have known for years: that we are in the midst of a profound and enduring birth control crisis that is unlikely to be resolved in this century. Yet the public still harbors the illusion that if the perfect contraceptive doesn't exist in the here and now, its development is imminent. This belief is so deeply ingrained that a 1985 Harris poll conducted

* Testimony presented at FDA hearings on the Vimule cervical cap, Rockville, Md., Sept. 13–14, 1984.

in the United States revealed that 76 percent of the adult population believe that a major breakthrough in contraceptive technology is likely within the next five years. *

A glance at current birth control research reveals only worse versions of the same old things—synthetic hormones implanted under the skin, tailless IUDs (intended primarily for use in the Third World), silicon plugs and a sort of intra-uterine glue designed to block the entrance to the egg tubes, and more widespread use of permanent surgical sterilization. The unembellished truth is that there is not going to be a "perfect" contraceptive, at least in the foreseeable future. As for male birth control: even on the remote possibility that a safe, effective, hassle-free male method might be developed, the chances of getting men to use it reliably and in large numbers are slim to none. Men are simply not going to take some cockamamie injection that lowers libido, makes their hair fall out, and causes their testicles to shrink. They know they don't have to.

The upshot of the modern birth control revolution and the ensuing crisis is that, in an age that offers remarkable sexual freedom, while demanding at the same time enormous sexual responsibility, women and their partners face a dwindling number of contraceptive options.

THE BIRTH CONTROL CRISIS

The causes of the modern birth control crisis are neither mysterious nor inexplicable:

• *An unbridled legal system* which generates exorbitant costs in prosecuting or defending claims and routinely seeks astronomical awards, has precipitated a crisis in malpractice and liability insurance for researchers and manufacturers and has virtually broken the back of new contraceptive research and development. The cervical cap is a case in point. Dr. Koch estimates that it will cost $750,000 in malpractice pre-

---

* Louis Harris and Associates, "Public Attitudes About Sex Education, Family Planning and Abortion in the United States," Aug.–Sept. 1985.

miums to test his new cap models, and is contemplating overseas trials.

• *The paltry amount of funding* allocated to the development of new birth control alternatives is another problem. While the arms race careens ahead to the tune of $34 million an hour, a miserly $55 million—the bulk of it from public and private agencies in the United States—is spent worldwide on birth control research each year. A mere $4 million is allocated to investigating low-risk barrier methods. Ironically, because of the legal and regulatory crisis, almost none of the products of this research are ever likely to reach the U.S. marketplace.

• *Because of the way that the FDA has chosen to interpret the Device Amendments*—by placing all new contraceptive devices in the "significant risk" category—it is now exceedingly difficult to get even low-risk methods, like the cervical cap, approved for general use. (See pages 30–37 for a discussion of the cap's tortuous journey through the federal review process.)

• *The focus of the population control establishment* on high technology and its lack of attention to low-risk barrier methods is another major element in the birth control crisis.

Solutions
Toward the prospect of effecting meaningful changes in the legal system and in a firmly entrenched social order that values defense and corporate profits above the health and well-being of its populace, some solutions have been suggested.

To start with, some tentative steps have been taken to alleviate the legal crisis through state or Congressional limits on lawyers' contingency fees and a cap on damages for "pain and suffering." Yet consumer advocates point out the need for powerful legal deterrents, citing drug companies' past abuses, such as the aggressive and indiscriminate marketing of high-dose birth control Pills and the Dalkon Shield. Consumer groups have also suggested that the demand for safer products and more responsible marketing programs would force manufacturers to police themselves somewhat, and thus lower the risk of law suits and high damages.*

As those who have tried know all too well, reordering social priorities is easier said than done. Yet reining in the defense budget and focusing more of our resources on human needs seems essential if we are to avoid crises similar to the one that has occurred in the field of contraception in other areas of health care and social welfare. If scientists can send people to the moon and if space age computer technology can almost literally make angels dance on the head of a pin, why can't we have safe, effective birth control?

In regard to the FDA's view of all birth control devices as "significant risk," it has also been suggested that health and consumer groups seek to influence the Agency's treatment of specific products, so that low-risk items are not necessarily held to the same standards as heart pacemakers, artificial hearts, and other internal implants. While no one is advocating watering down Federal drug and device regulations, some critics have objected to the arbitrary classification of *all* new birth control drugs or devices as "significant risk" and question the Agency's definition of "significant risk" as "pregnancy."

ARE HIGH-TECH METHODS THE ANSWER?

Longtime birth control researchers Malcolm Potts and Robert Wheeler examined the birth control crisis in a 1981 article in *Family Planning Perspectives* entitled "The Quest for a Magic Bullet." Regarding the pitiful state of the art, they observed that "the world spends as much on contraceptive research and development in one year as it spends in 20 minutes on the arms race." They go on to ponder the philosophical implications of the current focus on very effective methods which have significant risks and high discontinuation rates and wonder if these methods ultimately offer a better success rate than less effective, low-risk options which have good continuation rates.

* Michele Galen, "Birth Control Options Limited by Litigation," *The National Law Journal*, October 20, 1986, p. 26.

These two old hands on the birth control scene conclude, "It may be useful to consider whether contraceptive research is being asked to do something that is impossible, namely, to produce a reversible, highly effective contraceptive free from side effects." They conclude that researchers and family-planning providers might do well to look more closely at combinations of less popular methods where contraceptive responsibility is shared by both partners.

Perhaps instead of looking for the mythical "one-shot" solution to our contraceptive problems, we might do well to focus on the one factor that could make any birth control method, especially low-risk methods, more effective: fertility awareness. From a research point of view, if we marshaled our energy toward *understanding* the menstrual cycle, instead of incessantly trying to *eliminate* it—at great profit to the drug companies—the future of birth control might not look so grim.

THE MODERN BIRTH CONTROL REVOLUTION

In the first decade of the modern birth control revolution, much of the interest focused on effectiveness and convenience, and henceforth all contraceptive drugs and devices came to be judged by the "effectiveness and convenience standard." Since 1960, when the Pill was first marketed, followed shortly by the IUD, an entire generation of young women has come of age assuming that highly effective, hassle-free birth control is their birthright—if not their reality.

The second decade of the birth control revolution saw the rise and fall of the Dalkon Shield. The women's health movement, investigative journalists, and dedicated consumer advocates exposed unethical research and marketing practices that allowed the Shield's manufacturer, A. H. Robins, to peddle its deadly device, but not before at least eighteen women had died unnecessarily, and many had suffered traumatic physical injuries, which frequently resulted in infertility. In the wake of the Dalkon Shield debacle, Congress enacted the Medical Device Amendments requiring thorough testing and reporting of clinical and laboratory data before approval of new medical devices, including those used for birth control. Feminist groups and health activists also focused intense scrutiny on the systemic effects of synthetic hormones and demanded that more thoroughgoing user education and screening be done by family-planning providers.

In spite of the lion's share of contraceptive research money going to high-technology methods, in the third decade of the birth control crisis the picture has begun to change. Pill use dropped 20 percent between 1970 and 1980. Because of a flurry of lawsuits, the manufacture of the IUD was abruptly discontinued and became for all practical purposes a non-method overnight. Due to the outbreak of AIDS and widespread prevalence of herpes and other sexually transmissible diseases, the condom is currently undergoing a dramatic rehabilitation, and the diaphragm has likewise experienced a modest comeback. Although it is not well documented, alternative health practitioners report an increasing interest in fertility awareness, withdrawal, and forms of sexual activity that keep the penis out of the vagina.

CHOOSING A BIRTH CONTROL METHOD

Choosing a birth control method, or changing to a new one, can be an agonizing process. Sometimes your decision may be based on the advice of a friend or made on the unquestioned recommendation of your doctor, but a truly informed decision involves far more than simply evaluating the known positives and negatives of any method. The risks and benefits need to be weighed against those of other appropriate and available methods and then evaluated against your own individual needs, preferences and habits.

If you are in a stable relationship you may want to consult your partner and take his preferences into consideration. If you do not have a steady partner, your decision may be predicated on how frequently you are able to find one. If you are looking for a new partner, and have to do quite a bit of "shopping around," you may be concerned that certain methods are too awkward to be used on a first date, do not offer sufficient protection against sexually transmissible diseases, or you may not have enough information to minimize certain inconveniences. If you are at the end of your rope and are contemplating surgical sterilization, or your partner is considering vasectomy, you may want to review all of your options one more time. In making birth control choices, it is important to realize that once your decision is made, it may not be final. What may be an appropriate option *now* might not be suitable in five or six years when you may have different goals, a different partner, or a different health condition—or when you have had a child.

The following survey is intended to help you make an informed choice about the cervical cap and other available methods of contraception. It may also be useful if you cannot be fit for a cap and have to decide on a new method or need to continue with your old one. Perhaps your partner will also find it informative. In addition, it might be useful for young women who are choosing contraception for the first time and are unfamiliar with the advantages, disadvantages, and risks of each method. In this somewhat arbitrary order of presentation, the diaphragm and the Today™ contraceptive sponge are listed immediately after the cervical cap because they are its nearest cousins and will be most often compared to it.

PRENTIF CAP IN ALL FOUR SIZES

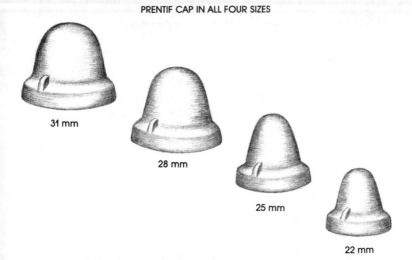

31 mm

28 mm

25 mm

22 mm

✳ THE CERVICAL CAP ✳ ✳ ✳ ✳ ✳ ✳ ✳ ✳

EFFECTIVENESS*

- Theoretical Effectiveness 98%
- Use Effectiveness 71%–98%
- Typical-User Effectiveness 83%

HEALTH RISKS

- None.

HEALTH BENEFITS

- You will be far less likely to contract sexually transmissible diseases, especially gonorrhea and chlamydia.
- You will be less likely to get pelvic inflammatory disease (PID) than women who do not use contraceptives.
- You may be protected from cervical cancer.

ADVANTAGES

- Can be left in place for several days at a time, offering prolonged protection while freeing one from the annoyance of interrupted sex.
- Uses only small amount of spermicide and is therefore less messy.
- Only needs to be used when sex is anticipated.

DISADVANTAGES

- Limited sizes, so not all women can be fit.
- Requires consistent and proper use to be effective.
- A few women find insertion and removal difficult.
- Your partner may experience some discomfort.
- Some women experience odor build-up after two to three days of use.

IMPACT ON FERTILITY

- Protects fertility.

* Most effectiveness rates are from *Contraceptive Technology*.

IMPACT ON SEXUALITY

- Does not interfere with sexual spontaneity.
- Does not interfere with sexual sensations.
- Not messy.
- Does not interfere with oral sex (see AIDS Warning below).
- Many cap users experience increased libido and increased frequency of sex.
- Can sometimes be uncomfortable for you or your partner.

AIDS Warning In view of the AIDS epidemic, it is now recommended that heterosexual couples avoid oral sex if they have

(1) had a recent change in partners;

(2) multiple partners;

or

(3) partner(s) with unknown sexual history.

In these circumstances, the use of condoms, dental dams or other rubber barriers is recommended.

Nonoxynol-9, the sperm-killing ingredient in most spermicides manufactured in the United States, has been found to kill the AIDS virus in laboratory tests. Whether or not it does so in "real life" remains to be proven. Nonetheless, using products containing nonoxynol-9, such as Ramses-Extra condoms and Foreplay and Lubraceptic lubricants, may offer some protection.*

* Personal communication, P. Clay Stephens, Fenway Clinic, Boston, Massachusetts.

MOST SUCCESSFUL USERS

- Women who use consistently and correctly.
- Women who have good insertion and removal skills.
- Women with confidence in the cap's effectiveness.

You should probably not use the cervical cap if
- you or your partner have an allergy to rubber or spermicide. (Some women choose to use the cap without spermicide and use a back-up method during their fertile times.)
- you cannot learn correct insertion and removal of the cap.
- you are uncomfortable touching your genitals.

COST FOR ONE YEAR
- $140, including fitting, lab fees, and spermicide.*

* THE DIAPHRAGM   * * * * * * * * *

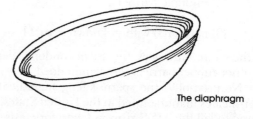

The diaphragm

The diaphragm has been humorously, and sometimes disparagingly, referred to by the post-Pill generation as "the old rubber parachute," "a dinghy for spermicide," "a Model-T Ford," "a flying saucer," and "a Frisbee," among other things. Yet this tried-and-true barrier method of birth control has served women admirably for more than a century.

The diaphragm was invented by Dr. C. Hasse, a German anatomy professor, in 1882, more than four decades after the cervical cap. For reasons that are not entirely clear, Hasse adopted the pseudonym Wilhelm P. J. Mensinga and marketed the device under that name. The diaphragm achieved modest popularity in its native Germany but came into its own in Holland in the 1880s, where it was often provided by midwives and shopkeepers in back rooms, as well as by physicians

---

* All costs for prescriptive methods are based on $100 for a visit with a doctor and $25 for tests. Costs for supplies are based on having intercourse three times a week. Costs for a clinic visit and supplies may be half as much.

and their assistants in formal birth control clinics. By the time Margaret Sanger visited Holland in 1915, the diaphragm was widely used and was known as the "Mensinga pessary." In England, it became known as the "Dutch cap." (These terms are a continuing source of confusion. "Mensinga pessary" and "Dutch cap" refer to the diaphragm. "Check pessary" refers to the cervical cap.)

Initially the cervical cap and the diaphragm were both used with homemade spermicides of questionable effectiveness and it was not until the late 1920s that reliable commercial spermicides, made from lactic acid and glycerine, were universally available and recommended. By now, most practitioners have come to accept the idea that the diaphragm has a dual function—that it acts both as a barrier and as a receptacle to hold spermicide against the cervix. Some even hold a minority view, suggesting that it is *primarily* a spermicidal container.

One of the most commonly voiced complaints about the diaphragm is that it can cause discomfort or pain after being worn for even a few hours. While a good deal of research has been done on diaphragm effectiveness, little attention has been devoted to this crucial issue.

The "largest is best" philosophy of cap fitting seems to have been developed by Dr. Dorothy Bocker, the first director of the Margaret Sanger clinic. This method of fitting, which depended on the distance between the pubic bone and the back of the vagina, and required spermicide, was in opposition to the European method, described by Robert Latou Dickinson in 1924, which called for a small diaphragm placed directly over the cervix and held in place by the vaginal muscles— similar to the way the Dumas cap is used today. In 1980, Dr. Edward Stim published a paper proposing a return to the "nonspermicide fit-free diaphragm," * and argued his case persuasively. Yet no one has attempted to duplicate his results, and large, painful diaphragms continue to be one of the major causes of discontinuation. The publication *Contraceptive*

---

* Edward M. Stim, "The Nonspermicide Fit-free Diaphragm," *Advances in Planned Parenthood* 15 (3), 1980.

Technology proposes that the device performs a dual function —both barrier and spermicidal holder.

Masters and Johnson, among the few researchers to explore the issue of diaphragm fit, found that even a well-fit diaphragm can buckle or gap during sexual activity—which may allow sperm to get over the rim—so a large size may be no better than a smaller, more comfortable one. While this research is not conclusive, it underlines the importance of using spermicide and adding it for repeated sessions of intercourse.

Over the years, women and their practitioners have come up with a number of "home remedies" which can help make diaphragm use more comfortable.

• If your diaphragm is uncomfortable or causes pain, don't hesitate to return to your practitioner and ask for a smaller one.

• To make the diaphragm less obtrusive in sex, insert it up to six hours ahead of time.

• If "post-coital drip" is bothersome, use light-day pads to catch any residue.

• Buy several diaphragms and keep one at home, one in the car, and one at your partner's house.

• The diaphragm can be used during your period to catch the menstrual flow, but should be removed after six to eight hours to avoid any risk of Toxic Shock Syndrome (see pages 88–89 for information on TSS).

• Try to incorporate use of the diaphragm into your sexual routine, eliciting your partner's cooperation and support.

• Have your partner purchase cream or jelly at times.

How to Use

Fill the dome with about a tablespoon of spermicidal cream or jelly and run a thin ribbon around the rim. Then fold the rim in half and insert it into the vagina with the open part toward the roof of the vagina. Push it as far back as it will go, until the front part of the rim hooks securely under the pubic bone. *Now check with your finger to see that the cervix is covered by the rubber dome.*

EFFECTIVENESS
- Theoretical Effectiveness 98%
- Use Effectiveness 81%–98%
- Typical-User Effectiveness 92%

HEALTH RISKS
- About 10 percent of diaphragm users experience repeated urinary-tract infections.

HEALTH BENEFITS
- You will be far less likely to contract sexually transmissible diseases such as gonorrhea, herpes, and trichomoniasis.
- You will be only half as likely to get pelvic inflammatory disease (PID) as women who do not use contraceptives.
- If you use the diaphragm for five years or more, you have about half the risk of getting cervical cancer.

ADVANTAGES
- Only needs to be used when sex is anticipated.
- Is low-risk.
- Protects against some sexually transmissible diseases.

DISADVANTAGES
- Must be used with every session of intercourse to be highly effective.
- Can be messy.
- Spermicide must be added for repeated sessions of intercourse.
- Must be left in place for six to eight hours.
- Can be painful if fit too large.
- If you have sex very often, spermicide requires constant resupply.

IMPACT ON FERTILITY
- Protects future fertility.

IMPACT ON SEXUALITY
- May interfere with spontaneity or sexual sensations.
- Some women who do not have steady partners find use awkward with new sexual partners.
- Use of spermicide increases vaginal lubrication.

- Must be inserted for each sexual encounter, but may be put in up to six hours ahead of anticipated intercourse.
- Spermicide can be messy and may make oral sex uncomfortable or less enjoyable. (See caution on oral sex and AIDS, page 121.)

MOST SUCCESSFUL USERS

- Women who use consistently and correctly.
- Women who have confidence in the diaphragm's effectiveness.

WHO SHOULD NOT USE

You should probably not use the diaphragm if
- you have repeated urinary-tract infections.
- you have allergies to rubber or spermicides.
- you have a pubic bone that is too shallow to hold the rim in place.
- you have certain anatomical conditions such as poor vaginal muscle tone, a cystocele, or a rectocele (protrusions of the bladder or rectum into the vagina).
- you have a history of Toxic Shock Syndrome.
- you are very uncomfortable touching your genitals.

COST FOR ONE YEAR

- $200, including fitting, lab fees, and spermicide.

✳ THE TODAY™ CONTRACEPTIVE SPONGE ✳ ✳ ✳

This synthetic update of the natural sea sponges of antiquity was marketed in 1983 by VLI, a California corporation, and quickly became "the leading over-the-counter contraceptive for women."* The Today™ contraceptive sponge comes in one size and looks like a dimpled marshmallow with a loop on its back (to aid removal). It works by releasing spermicide, absorbing the man's ejaculate, and blocking the entry of sperm into the cervical canal. The sponge, designed for one-time use, is suffused with almost twice as much nonoxynol-9 (10 percent) as is contained in most spermicidal creams or jellies.

* *Contraceptive Technology Update*, July 1985.

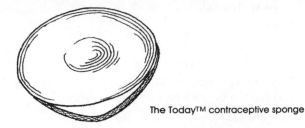

The Today™ contraceptive sponge

Some women have found that the sponge can flake or disintegrate in the vagina—making removal difficult and occasionally requiring medical help—and that it can slip during intercourse. Pregnancy rates have varied widely, and many are lower than those for other barrier methods. Some cases of Toxic Shock Syndrome (TSS) have been attributed to sponge use, but the Centers for Disease Control estimate that the chances of an individual woman developing TSS from sponge use are about a million to one, approximately the same as for using tampons. The developers, however, claim that the sponge inhibits the growth of staph *aureus*, the bacteria responsible for TSS. To reduce any risk of TSS, do not use sponges during menstrual bleeding and do not keep them in place for more than twenty-four hours. (For information on TSS, see pages 88–89.)

How to Use

Dampen the sponge, fold it slightly, and insert it into your vagina, turning it so that the dimple is facing toward the cervix, then check with your finger to see if it is correctly positioned. If you put it in quite a while before you have intercourse, it is a good idea to check placement just beforehand, as well as afterward, to make sure it hasn't slipped. If you find the sponge out of its expected place very often, make an appointment with your doctor or family-planning clinic to check your insertion technique and to determine if your vaginal muscles are strong enough to hold the sponge in place.

EFFECTIVENESS
- Use Effectiveness 72%–90%
- Typical-User Effectiveness 84%–87%

HEALTH RISKS
• None.

HEALTH BENEFITS
• May protect against some sexually transmitted diseases and cervical infections that can lead to cancer.

ADVANTAGES
• Can be purchased without a prescription.
• Less messy than the diaphragm.

DISADVANTAGES
• You or your partner may experience irritation or itching.
• Unless bought in large quantities, requires constant resupply.
• Can be difficult to remove, and occasionally shreds, leaving bits of sponge in the vagina.
• May develop an odor after intercourse.

IMPACT ON FERTILITY
• Protects fertility.

IMPACT ON SEXUALITY
• Does not interfere with spontaneity if inserted well ahead of time.
• May be felt by partner.
• May absorb vaginal secretions and cause dryness.
• Because the sponge absorbs ejaculate and does not have a liquid spermicide, there is less post-coital drip.
• Does not interfere with oral sex. (See cautions on oral sex and AIDS, page 121.)

MOST SUCCESSFUL USERS
• Women who use correctly and consistently.
• Women who do not want to use prescription items.
• Young women who may find it appealing because it is attractively packaged, available without a prescription, and easy to use.
• Women who have confidence in the sponge's effectiveness.

You should not use the sponge if
- you have a history of Toxic Shock Syndrome.
- you or your partner has an allergy to nonoxynol-9 or polyure-thane.
- you cannot learn correct insertion technique.

COST FOR ONE YEAR

- $70 for an average of one sponge per week @ $1.25 each.
  $210 for an average of three sponges a week @ $1.25 each.

✳ THE PILL ✳ ✳ ✳ ✳ ✳ ✳ ✳ ✳ ✳ ✳ ✳

Recipes for potions taken by mouth to prevent conception can be found in almost every culture, their composition ranging from the traditional Talmudic "cup of roots" to a catalog of both simple and bizarre concoctions covering the gamut of animal, vegetable, and mineral. While midwives, witch doctors and shamans swore by their prescriptions, history leaves a blank on the actual effectiveness of these libations. One could argue that the birth control Pill of today is yet another item in this colorful and inventive apothecary, but it differs significantly in one respect. Its formulation is based upon a scientific understanding, rudimentary though it may be, of the menstrual cycle.

In the 1930s, modern science began to acquire an understanding of the delicate interplay of hormones that results in the cyclic production of a viable egg in the ovary. In the late

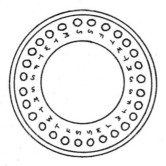

A Pill packet

1940s, Dr. Gregory Pincus, a Boston infertility researcher, and Dr. Min Cheuh Chang discovered that progesterone, manufactured by the ovary, actually had the power to inhibit conception—at least in rabbits. Then in the early 1950s, Dr. Russell Marker, a University of Pennsylvania chemist, isolated progesterone from Mexican wild yams and founded Syntex, a small drug company, to produce the product. But extracting the chemical from yams was an expensive process, so Dr. Carl Djerassi, a Syntex chemist, succeeded in making a cheaper compound which had a progesterone-like effect. Shortly thereafter, G. D. Searle patented a similar formula. The drug that these researchers developed suppresses normal hypothalamic/pituitary/ovarian function, short-circuiting the menstrual cycle and inhibiting the release of hormones which promote the cyclic maturation of an egg.

Margaret Sanger, who was forever on the watch for new contraceptive possibilities, threw her considerable support, and the money of tractor heiress Katherine Douglas McCormick, behind the research of Pincus and Dr. John Rock, an enterprising Harvard endocrinologist in the early 1950s. Pincus and Rock began trials with the Searle formula in Puerto Rico in 1956 and a mere four years later, in 1960, the modern birth control revolution had begun. In the succeeding quarter of a century, the Pill became the most widely used method of *reversible* contraception in the world.

Today, two types of Pills are available in the United States, *combined Pills*, containing both estrogen and progesterone, and progesterone-only *mini-pills*. The *triphasic Pill* is a type of combined Pill, providing decreasing doses of estrogen and an increased dose of progesterone as the cycle progresses. Triphasics are said to more closely mimic the normal menstrual cycle by providing an ever-increasing dose of progesterone in three incremental stages, but there is considerable controversy over whether this simulation of the menstrual cycle is truly advantageous.

Many women use the Pill successfully. In addition to the freedom from anxiety about pregnancy, they benefit from lessened premenstrual symptoms, less painful periods, and possibly decreased incidence of pelvic inflammatory disease caused by gonorrhea. Approximately fifteen percent of all users of the Pill take it for noncontraceptive reasons. Many women also experience a panoply of physical disorders, some of which remain after Pill use ceases, and a few incur serious, even life-threatening conditions. *Women who are 35 and smoke, or who are over 40, are definitely at higher risk for serious Pill-related complications.*

Note If you have been on the Pill for a long time and are still on higher-dose pills, and you haven't had any trouble, you may feel secure in continuing with your present prescription. However, *high-dosage pills, which were much more widely used in the past, are far more dangerous for women over thirty.* If you don't want to change your method, you should definitely ask your doctor to change your prescription to a lower-dose Pill, even if he or she doesn't suggest it.

The Pill may interfere with the absorption of some vitamins such as A, B-2, B-6, B-12, C and folic acid and may alter carbohydrate metabolism. When taken in combination with certain prescription drugs, especially phenobarbital and Dilantin, rifampin (used in the treatment of tuberculosis), anticonvulsants and some antibiotics, its ability to prevent pregnancy may be decreased. Conversely, oral contraceptives may significantly prolong the effects of Valium in the blood stream.

How to Use

The Pill in its various guises is praised for its convenience, yet there is more to proper use of this method than remembering to take a Pill every day. If you take oral contraceptives, you need to be aware of the commonly accepted Pill danger signs and return to your practitioner for evaluation if any occur. *Contraceptive Technology* has outlined the Pill danger signs with the easily remembered acronym ACHES.* If you are on the Pill and experience any of the following symptoms, contact your doctor or clinic *immediately*.

A = Abdominal pain (severe)

C = Chest pain (severe), cough, shortness of breath

H = Headache (severe), dizziness, weakness, numbness

E = Eye problems (vision loss or blurring), speech problems

S = Severe leg pain (calf or thigh)

EFFECTIVENESS

- Theoretical effectiveness: 99 + %
- Use effectiveness:
    - Combined Pills 99.5% (adults)
    - Mini-pills 98% (adults)
- Typical-user effectiveness:
    - Combined Pills 98% (adults)
    - Mini-pills 96% (adults)   94.5% (teenagers) †

HEALTH RISKS

Major Risks
- Blood clots
- Heart attack
- Stroke
- Benign liver tumors (hepatocellular adenomas, which while benign, can be fatal if they burst) and possibly liver cancer (hepatocellular carcinoma)
- High blood pressure
- Blurred vision or loss of vision

Less Serious, but Annoying, Pill Disorders
- Headaches
- Nausea
- Breakthrough bleeding
- Water retention (edema)
- Breast pain, tenderness, fullness or growth

* From *Contraceptive Technology*, 1986–1987. Used by permission.

† Includes both combined and mini-pills. Because many teenagers do not take their Pills exactly as prescribed, some practitioners are hesitant to prescribe the mini-pill, which should be taken at the same time every day to be effective.

- No bleeding at time of period
- Failure of menses to return after discontinuation of Pills
- Loss of sex drive (libido)
- Skin discoloration (cholasma)
- Acne
- Decreased vaginal lubrication
- Growth of fibroids
- Contact lenses may not fit correctly

Note Pill use does not appear to have any effect on the incidence of breast cancer, one way or another.

HEALTH BENEFITS

- You may experience less painful menstrual cramps, decreased pain from endometriosis and less severe pre-menstrual syndrome (PMS).
- Pill users have a lower risk of pelvic inflammatory disease (PID) caused by gonorrhea (but not by chlamydia). If you use the Pill for one year and have never had PID, you have only half the risk of contracting acute PID as women who are not using any form of birth control (except abstinence). The lowered risk lasts only as long as you take the Pill.
- You may have a lowered incidence of noncancerous cysts in the breast, but not of fibrous growths (fibroadenoma). The reduced risk of cystic breast conditions occurs after one to two years of Pill use and remains for about one year after discontinuation.
- Because your menstrual flow will be lighter, you will be about half as likely to develop iron-deficiency anemia as non-Pill users.
- Because the normal function of the ovary is suppressed, certain types of ovarian cysts and cellular changes are less likely to develop. You will be about 90 percent less likely to develop *functional* ovarian cysts (those related to ovulation) while the risk of *non-functional* ovarian cysts remains the same as for non-Pill users.
- Research data suggests that Pill users experience about one half the incidence of ovarian and endometrial cancer after one year of Pill use. Some researchers think that this effect may last a lifetime.

ADVANTAGES
- Highly effective.
- Easy to take.
- Use can be totally separated from sexual activity.

DISADVANTAGES
- Must be taken every day to be effective.
- Requires a prescription and follow-up visits.
- Requires constant resupply.
- May be expensive for some women.

IMPACT ON FERTILITY
- May protect against pelvic inflammatory disease caused by gonorrhea.
- Normal menstruation returns for most women within several months of discontinuing Pill use, but for some women conception can take up to two years to occur.

IMPACT ON SEXUALITY
- Sex is completely spontaneous.
- Vaginal lubrication may be less or take longer to occur.
- May decrease desire for sex. Not feeling well because of the Pill's effects on many body systems may also decrease interest in sex. "Not tonight, honey, I have a headache," may be the literal truth for some Pill users.

MOST SUCCESSFUL USERS
- Women who use correctly and consistently.
- Women who do not have debilitating Pill-related disorders.
- Women who are not afraid of short-term or long-term health risks of the Pill.

WHO SHOULD NOT USE
You should *absolutely not use the Pill* if you
- have a history of or current heart or liver disease, cancer of the reproductive organs, including breasts, uterus, and ovaries.
- are over 35 and smoke.
- might be pregnant.
- are a heavy user of alcohol or drugs.
- have a history of mental illness.

You should *seriously consider not using the Pill* if you have
• migraine or increasingly chronic headaches.
• high blood pressure.
• sickle cell disease.
• diabetes.

CONTINUATION RATE AFTER ONE YEAR
• 50–70%

COST FOR ONE YEAR
• $100–$150   for physician's visit and prescription and lab tests
• $115–$260   13 packets of Pills purchased at drug store
• $15–$115   13 packets of Pills purchased at clinic

✳ THE IUD   ✳ ✳ ✳ ✳ ✳ ✳ ✳ ✳ ✳ ✳ ✳ ✳

The first IUDs were probably stones inserted through hollow tubes into the uteruses of camels by migratory tribes at least two thousand years ago. Although few details are known, over the centuries women in various cultures may have inserted little balls made of glass, wood, or precious metals into their own uteruses. An early twentieth-century IUD made of a circle of silkworm gut and wire caused hideous infections and had a high failure rate. Current IUDs were developed in the United States in the 1960s, and the *Progestasert-T*, a progesterone-impregnated device, followed in the 1970s. The high

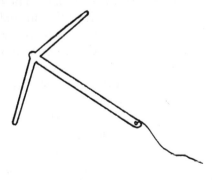

The Progestasert IUD

infection rate caused by IUDs has been attributed to the existence of the "tail," which offers bacteria a sort of ladder into the uterus. Tailless IUDs, which are widely used in China and in other parts of the world, have much lower infection rates, but much higher incidences of complications upon removal.

Following the discontinuation of the Saf-T-Coil in 1985 by its manufacturer, Julius Schmid, Ortho Pharmaceuticals announced that it would no longer manufacture the Lippes Loop. Shortly thereafter, G. D. Searle, faced with a spate of lawsuits, announced the discontinuation of the Copper-7. The companies readily admitted that they were motivated by the fear of litigation over injuries suffered by IUD users.

Even before its disappearance from the U.S. market, IUD use in Planned Parenthood clinics declined significantly. In 1970, 15.3 percent of new clients requested the IUD, but by 1980, only 4.5 percent did.

Exactly how the IUD prevents pregnancy is still something of a mystery. It may make the uterus inhospitable to the implantation of a fertilized egg by creating an inflammation inside of the uterus, or the tail may introduce bacteria which cause a low-grade infection. It may dislodge an implanted egg or cause expulsion of a fertilized egg by stimulating the production of prostaglandins, a substance that causes uterine contractions. Or, through some unknown mechanism, the IUD may cause the egg tubes to vibrate faster than normal and expel the egg before it can be fertilized. (Eggs are normally fertilized in the upper part of the egg tube.) The copper in copper-bearing IUDs may adversely affect the normal intrauterine ecology in several ways, and the synthetic progestin in the Progestasert IUD may thicken fertile mucus enough to block the entry of the sperm into the cervical canal. It is possible that any one or a combination of these factors may be responsible for the IUD's effectiveness.

The only IUD remaining on the U.S. market today is the Progestasert-T. This device, which releases synthetic progesterone into the bloodstream by osmosis, has not been favored by practitioners, partly because it must be replaced every year and partly because "adding hormones to IUDs only adds another set of potential side effects to those already existing," as Betsy Hartmann, author of *Reproductive Rights and Wrongs*,* observes. It remains to be seen how popular the Progestasert-T will be now that it is the only IUD available. Because Planned Parenthood has a policy of providing all approved methods of birth control, the Progestasert will be available in all of its clinics.

Although much has been made over the IUD's potential to cause infertility, it is now thought that women who do not have multiple partners can use IUDs with relative safety—*if neither of the couple has sex outside of their relationship.* In this regard, as Shere Hite documented in *The Hite Report*, an estimated 70 percent of men and 50 percent of women do have sex outside of their primary relationships, at least occasionally, and do not usually divulge such activity to their partners.

Expulsion of the IUD may occur in up to 20 percent of users in the first year. The device can also become embedded in the uterine wall, or occasionally "migrate" through the wall into the pelvic cavity. Keeping regular tabs on your string is the best defense against these complications.

IUD users who take antibiotics are more likely to get pregnant, possibly because the drug clears up a low-grade infection created by the device in the uterus. Therefore, it is highly advisable to use a back-up method, like foam and/or condoms, or to keep the penis out of the vagina during antibiotic treatment and for a few weeks afterward. In general, use of a back-up method is recommended for the first three months of IUD use, since higher incidences of pregnancy and expulsion occur during this time. Women are seldom informed that plastic IUDs are impregnated with a small amount of radioactive barium to make the device more visible on X-rays.

FDA standards now allow IUDs, including copper devices, to remain in place for up to four years if no problems arise, and many women who already have them will continue to use them. Since IUDs are not illegal, only unavailable,

---

* Betsy Hartmann, *Reproductive Rights and Wrongs: The Global Politics of Population Control and Contraceptive Choice* (New York: Harper & Row, 1987).

some doctors and clinics may have stockpiles that could last for several years. So if you really want one, ask around. Some women who live in states bordering Canada, and even in New York, are apparently traveling to Canada to get the devices inserted.

How to Use

The primary advantage of the IUD is that it is unlikely to be forgotten or misused. Proper use, however, requires you to check the string frequently at first, then monthly after your period. A missing string may mean that the IUD has become embedded or passed through the uterine wall, or that it has been expelled. Many feminist clinics will give you a plastic speculum and show you how to check for the string visually with one—a much more direct way to keep tabs on it.

You also need to be aware of any sign of a problem and call your practitioner *immediately* if any one of them develops. If you are traveling, *do not wait until you return home* to call a practitioner. If you get pregnant with the IUD in place, the chances of miscarriage are about 50 percent.

The IUD danger signs are:

P = Period late (pregnancy), abnormal spotting or bleeding
A = Abdominal pain, pain with intercourse
I = Infection exposure (such as gonorrhea), abnormal discharge
N = Not feeling well, fever, chills
S = String missing, shorter or longer *

EFFECTIVENESS
• Theoretical Effectiveness 98.5%
• Use Effectiveness 90%–96%
• Typical-User Effectiveness 95%

---

* From *Contraceptive Technology*, 1986–87. Used by permission.

- Abnormal bleeding, hemorrhage, or anemia.
- Uterine perforation upon insertion or embedding in uterine wall or migration into abdominal cavity.
- Two to ten times higher incidence of PID than women who do not use IUDs. PID can become chronic and result in infertility, ectopic pregnancy, inflammation of the uterine lining (endometritis).

Note According to *Contraceptive Technology*, when PID is diagnosed the IUD should be removed before treatment begins, and if pregnancy is confirmed and an infection is present, the IUD should be removed at once to avoid a potentially fatal infection (sepsis) that can cross the placenta and enter the bloodstream.

HEALTH BENEFITS

- The only health benefit of the IUD is decreased menstrual bleeding from elimination of the menstrual cycle caused by the Progestasert, which is infused with the same synthetic hormone —progestin—as the mini-pill.

ADVANTAGES

- Highly effective.
- Cannot be misused.
- Does not interfere with sexual spontaneity.

DISADVANTAGES

- Heavier, crampier periods for some women, resulting in greater blood loss and possible anemia.

IMPACT ON FERTILITY

- If you have multiple partners, or you or your partner have sex with others, you may have up to ten times the risk of infertility that non–IUD users have. If you are monogamous you have a two percent higher incidence of infertility.

- If you want to have children in the future, you should seriously consider using another method.

IMPACT ON SEXUALITY
- Does not interfere with sexual spontaneity.
- Infrequently, partners can feel the string, which may cause chafing or scratches on the penis.

MOST SUCCESSFUL USERS
- Couples who do not have sex with others.
- Women who do not want children in the future.
- Women who have had at least one previous birth.

WHO SHOULD NOT USE
You should not use the IUD if you
- have a current pelvic infection.
- have an acute or chronic cervical infection.
- have an abnormal Pap smear.
- have a history of tubal pregnancy.
- have many sexual partners.
- have diabetes, sickle-cell disease, anemia.
- think you might be pregnant.

COST FOR ONE YEAR
- $200 Progestasert, including physician visit, insertion, and follow-up. (Does not include cost if IUD use results in hospitalization for PID or if it must be removed surgically.) If you have the same device for three or four years, the annual cost is only $40 or $50.

✳ SURGICAL STERILIZATION FOR WOMEN ✳ ✳ ✳

The first surgical sterilization was performed in the United States in 1880 as an alternative to removing the ovaries to prevent further pregnancies in a woman having her second cesarean birth. In the next three quarters of a century, some surgical sterilizations were done as major surgery under general anesthesia, but the practice was generally discouraged because of surgical complications and long hospital stays.

With the perfection of the laparoscope in the late 1960s, direct visualization of the abdominal cavity became possible, making surgical sterilization a much simpler procedure appropriate for a clinical setting using only local anesthesia.

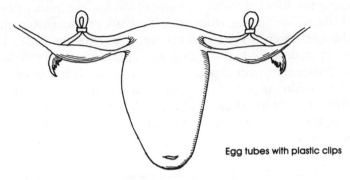

Egg tubes with plastic clips

Surgical sterilization, used by about 15 million women and men in the United States, is commonly referred to as our "most popular" method of contraception. But the use of the term "popular" is misleading. Many people do not so much *choose* sterilization as *resort* to it when there are no amenable alternatives. For some, who resort to surgery under extreme duress, even the term *voluntary* presses the point. It might be more appropriate to refer to surgical sterilization as our *most widely used method.*

Many variant methods of surgical sterilization have been developed, but today only two types are widely used throughout the world. In *laparoscopy*, the abdominal cavity is inflated with gas and the laparoscope, a tube with a light attached, is inserted through an incision just below the belly button. A second instrument is then introduced to crush, clip or cauterize the tubes. In the less complicated *minilaparotomy* the laparoscope is inserted through a small incision, euphemistically called a "bikini cut," just above the pubic hairline. A major advantage of the minilap procedure is that gas inflation of the abdomen is not required.

Some tubal sterilizations do indeed "tie" the egg tubes with surgical-grade thread, but other methods for blocking them are clipping, ringing with plastic, and burning or crushing. Sterilization can also be done vaginally, leaving no visible scar, but complication rates are higher than for abdominal procedures. No method has outstanding advantages over the other, but organ damage from burning in electrocautery procedures can occur. New microsurgical techniques make repairing the tubes possible in some cases; but pregnancy does not always result. *Contraceptive Technology* warns that the published reversal rates of 50 percent to 70 percent may be gravely misleading because they are reported by highly skilled microsurgeons who operate only on carefully screened clients. Regret is one of the primary disadvantages of the procedure. One study shows that more than one million couples regret their decisions and would take advantage of reversal if it were available.*

Note You should think of surgical sterilization as permanent and irreversible.

EFFECTIVENESS

- Theoretical Effectiveness 99.95%
- Use Effectiveness 99.92%–99.96%

HEALTH RISKS

- From one to ten women in one hundred thousand die from anesthesia-related complications.
- About one percent of women who are sterilized experience surgical complications such as shock, infection, post-operative bleeding, uterine perforation, and damage to bowel, bladder, or other organs during surgery.
- Post-surgical complications include a rare tubal pregnancy, menstrual irregularities (increased or decreased flow), and chronic pelvic pain.

* Linda E. Atkinson, Richard Lincoln, and Jacqueline Darroch Forrest, "The Next Contraceptive Revolution," *Family Planning Perspectives*, vol. 18, no. 1 (Jan.–Feb. 1986), p. 20.

HEALTH BENEFITS
• None.

ADVANTAGES
• Complete sexual spontaneity.
• No ongoing expense.
• Can't be misused.

DISADVANTAGES
• Expensive, unless you have insurance.
• Permanent in most cases. If life circumstances change, you may regret your decision.
• No protection against sexually transmissible diseases.

IMPACT ON FERTILITY
• Fertility is intentionally and permanently eliminated.

IMPACT ON SEXUALITY
• Complete spontaneity.

MOST SUCCESSFUL USERS
• Women who want no future children.
• Women who do not have personal or cultural objections to being sterile.

WHO SHOULD NOT USE
• Young women.
• Women who may want children in the future.
• Women whose feelings about marriage, commitment, and raising a family are unclear.

COST FOR ONE YEAR
• $2,000, including doctor's fee and anesthesiologist. (Does not include cost of surgical complications.) Cost spread out over many years makes sterilization as cheap as other methods.

Nineteenth-century European surgeons sometimes performed effective vasectomies in conjunction with prostate surgery to reduce post-operative swelling, and the procedure was occasionally performed on criminals and mental patients for contraceptive purposes in the United States in the early twentieth century. The procedure was first used on a wide scale in Bangladesh and India in the 1950s and 1960s. According to *Population Reports,** "vasectomy received a major boost when adverse publicity about the oral contraceptive coincided with a feminist campaign to encourage greater male responsibility in reproduction." Today, about half a million men in the U.S. decide to undergo—or resort to—"the snip" each year.

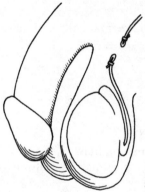

Severed vas deferens in vasectomy

Vasectomy is a twenty-minute outpatient procedure which requires one or two small incisions in the scrotal sac. The twin parallel tubes of the vas deferens are cut, then crushed and tied or clipped, or burned with a small electrode. None of these procedures appears to have marked advantages, but ones that destroy less of the tubes may have a better chance for reattachment later. Most physicians recommend

* Judith Wortman and P. T. Piotrow, "Vasectomy: Old and New Techniques," *Population Reports* (Series D, no. 1, December, 1973).

taking it easy for two or three days after the procedure, and suggest foregoing intercourse for a week to ten days to allow the vas to heal without stress.

The most perplexing issue associated with vasectomy is the development of sperm antibodies in response to leakage of sperm into the bloodstream which occurs in some men who have had the procedure, but researchers are unable to find any definable health risk associated with this phenomenon. No deaths from vasectomy have been reported in the United States, but a few occur worldwide each year.

It is possible to reattach the vas deferens, but success rates vary widely, depending upon the skill of the microsurgeon and several other factors, including type of procedure originally employed and length of time since the operation.

Note Vasectomy does not result in immediate sterility. It may take up to twenty ejaculations to clear the vas deferens of sperm. Men should use condoms or have their partners use a back-up method of birth control until they have a clear sperm count six to eight weeks after the procedure.

EFFECTIVENESS

- Theoretical Effectiveness 99.85%
- Use Effectiveness 97.8–99.9%

HEALTH RISKS

- Short-term: pain, burning, swelling (epididymitis), or infection.
- Long-term: development of abscesses or inflammation, hematoma (blood clot), infection up to six months after procedure.
- Infections require antibiotic treatment, and occasionally blood clots and swelling must be repaired surgically.

HEALTH BENEFITS

- None.

- Inexpensive and is frequently covered by insurance.
- Highly effective, easy to use, and use can be totally separated from intercourse.
- Men assume responsibility for birth control.
- May offer woman partner limited protection from some sexually transmitted diseases because no sperm enter vagina.

DISADVANTAGES

- Permanent in most cases. If life circumstances change, some men may regret their decisions.
- Men have no protection against sexually transmissible diseases and women have only limited protection.

IMPACT ON FERTILITY

- Fertility is effectively curtailed.

IMPACT ON SEXUALITY

- Allows for complete sexual spontaneity.
- Does *not* interfere with a man's sexual ability.

MOST SUCCESSFUL USERS

- Men who do not want future children.
- Men who have come to terms with their feelings about marriage, family, and committed relationships.
- Men who want to take responsibility for contraception.
- Men who do not have personal or cultural objections to being sterile.

WHO SHOULD NOT USE

- Teenagers.
- Men who may want future children.
- Men who are unsure of their feelings concerning marriage, family, and committed relationships.

COST

- $250–$300, including doctor's fee and follow-up. (Does not include cost for post-operative complications.) Spread over several years, cost is cheaper than most birth control methods.

✳ THE CONDOM ✳ ✳ ✳ ✳ ✳ ✳ ✳ ✳ ✳ ✳

During the Renaissance, linen sheaths for the penis were thought to prevent the transmission of syphilis, but their effectiveness for this purpose is highly questionable. Casanova was an early advocate of penile covers made from animal intestines for use as contraception, but it was not until the vulcanization of rubber in the 1840s that condoms became widely available. Although several intriguing theories have been put forward, the origin of the name "condom" remains a mystery.

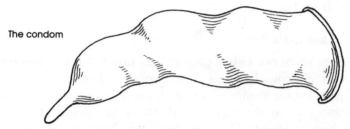

The condom

Today, condoms come in an ever-expanding variety of colors and textures, and are the second most widely used method of birth control in the world after surgical sterilization, with Japan and China accounting for nearly half of the world's use. In Western countries, condoms usually come in one size only, but recently some U.S. manufacturers have begun making more sizes. In China and Japan, condoms are made in three sizes to accommodate normal anatomical diversity and are thinner than Western brands. In the United States one brand of condom, the Ramses Extra, is now infused with nonoxynol-9, theoretically enhancing protection against pregnancy and sexually transmissible diseases, including AIDS.

Note Laboratory tests have shown that the AIDS virus does not pass through rubber condoms. However, *the popular condoms made from sheep-gut do not protect against AIDS.*

Many people associate condoms with illicit sex or extra-marital sexual activity and are resistant to buying them in a drugstore to use at home. Yet condoms are one of the cheapest, most effective and widely available birth control methods. "Sheaths," as they are also called, are commonly thought of as a male method, but it might be more appropriate to consider them a "joint" method, since it takes the consent of both partners to use them, and women can purchase them and suggest their use as readily as a man can. In Japan, where the condom is the method of choice, putting it on the penis has become an important part of sex play and its use is considered highly erotic.

How to Use

Before insertion, either partner can unroll the condom onto the erect penis. In a report on condoms, *Population Reports* explores some common assumptions about condom use and suggests some alternative methods of use that might make them more acceptable to some people.* It is usually recommended that the man remove the sheathed penis from the vagina right after ejaculation to avoid having any sperm seep out at the base of the penis, but the report suggests that this need not be done as long as the unrolled edge is held tightly against the base of the penis. There is also continuing controversy about whether or not sperm are in the lubricating fluid that seeps out of the penis shortly after erection. But in order to be protected against pregnancy *and* sexually transmitted diseases, it is best to put on the condom before insertion. The report also dismisses the idea that a space needs to be left at the tip in condoms that do not have reservoirs at the end to catch the ejaculate, noting that the rubber is highly elastic and should expand upon ejaculation.

It is often recommended that condoms be used in conjunction with foam or suppositories for "99 percent effectiveness," but, since condoms alone are highly effective when

* Jacqueline D. Sherris, Dana Lewison, and Gordon Fox, "Update on Condoms: Products, Protection, Promotion," *Population Reports* (Series H, no. 6, Sept.–Oct. 1982).

used regularly and correctly, the authors of *Population Reports* wonder if the extra trouble and expense is worth a few points of effectiveness and if it perhaps discourages use.

Condoms come in both lubricated and nonlubricated versions. If you find that you still need more lubrication, try K-Y Jelly or other water-based lubricants. The use of petroleum jelly is no longer recommended, since it is an oil-based product that can damage the thin rubber of the condom and may be absorbed through the vaginal walls as well.

EFFECTIVENESS

• Theoretical Effectiveness 98%–99%
• Use Effectiveness 90%–98.4%
• Typical-User Effectiveness 96%

> **Note** The Ramses Extra brand of condoms, infused with nonoxynol-9, has been found to be highly effective in killing sperm (on the inside of the condom).

HEALTH RISKS

• None.

HEALTH BENEFITS

• Offers both women and men the best protection against sexually transmissible diseases including gonorrhea, syphilis, herpes, chlamydia, and AIDS.
• Protects the cervix against pre-cancerous conditions.

ADVANTAGES

• Highly effective.
• Offers best protection against sexually transmissible diseases.
• Widely available.
• Convenient to carry.
• Inexpensive.

DISADVANTAGES
- Must be used consistently to be effective.
- Requires consent of both partners.
- One size does not necessarily fit all.
- Can occasionally leak or burst during use—visually checking condoms for leaks, and not reusing, can help minimize this problem. Blowing them up to check for leaks is no longer recommended—it can stretch and damage the rubber.

IMPACT ON FERTILITY
- Protects future fertility.

IMPACT ON SEXUALITY
- Intercourse is less messy because the condom catches the ejaculate.
- May reduce sexual sensation for some people.
- May be difficult to use if the man is not able to predict ejaculation.
- Some young people find using condoms awkward, especially on initial sexual encounters.
- An excellent back-up or emergency method of birth control.

MOST SUCCESSFUL USERS
- Individuals or couples who use condoms correctly and consistently.
- Couples with good communication about sex.
- Individuals or couples who want protection against sexually transmissible diseases.

WHO SHOULD NOT USE
- People with allergies to rubber.
- Men who have difficulty controlling erection.

CONTINUATION RATE AFTER ONE YEAR
- Continuation rates vary quite a bit depending upon age, motivation, and future fertility plans.

• $20, based on use of one to two a week.

✳ SPERMICIDAL FOAM AND SUPPOSITORIES   ✳ ✳

Spermicidal agents have been used alone or in combination with pessaries, sponges, or tampons throughout history. The ancient Egyptians employed a mixture of honey and sodium carbonate, which probably immobilized sperm as well as killed it. Updated nineteenth-century versions featured a variety of agents, including boric acid, lactic acid, and quinine sulfate in a base of cocoa butter or glycerine. Homegrown remedies are still used in many parts of the world and even in the United States where some women report that they make their own using lemon juice in a base of aloe vera gel.

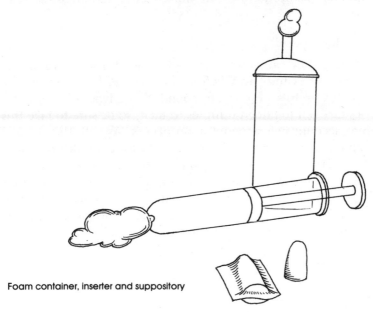

Foam container, inserter and suppository

Major advances in the composition of spermicidal agents occurred in the 1950s with the introduction of foaming suppositories, aerosol containers, and new chemical formulas.

Today, there are more than twenty-five types of vaginal spermicides manufactured worldwide, including foam, jelly, cream, and suppositories. Most contain nonoxynol-9 as the spermicidal agent, but only a few of them are available in the United States. Suppositories are especially popular in Germany, even among young women, and in Japan and other Asian countries as well, where an aggressive marketing campaign is helping the Neo Sampoon suppository gain acceptance.

Spermicides—especially when used in conjunction with condoms, the diaphragm, or the cervical cap—are highly effective and are extremely low-risk. Because of their protection against sexually transmissible diseases and ready availability, spermicidal foam and suppositories ought to be more heavily promoted as a viable option, but many family-planning practitioners do not present them in a favorable light, conveying the impression that they are not effective and are difficult to use.

How to Use

Because they can run, most women don't insert foam or gel suppositories until just before intercourse, but they can be inserted up to an hour beforehand. Some types of suppositories take ten to fifteen minutes to melt, so be sure to take this into account before penetration occurs. As with the cervical cap and diaphragm, it is important to have an idea of where your cervix is, so that you can place the applicator of foam or the suppository right next to it. A new suppository or another applicator must be used for repeated sessions of intercourse. Aerosol cans tend to run out unexpectedly, so it is a good idea always to keep an extra one on hand.

EFFECTIVENESS
• Theoretical Effectiveness 95%–97%
• User Effectiveness 71%–98.5%
• Typical-User Effectiveness 87%

HEALTH RISKS
• None.

HEALTH BENEFITS

• Protection against sexually transmitted diseases, including herpes and trichomoniasis, and pelvic inflammatory disease caused by gonorrhea and chlamydia.

ADVANTAGES

• Does not require a prescription.
• Can be used as an occasional or interim method or as back-up with other methods during fertile time.
• Men can buy and take responsibility for birth control.

DISADVANTAGES

• Must be used properly every time to be highly effective.
• Suppositories need to be inserted a few minutes prior to intercourse and thus require partner cooperation.
• Some couples view spermicides and suppositories as messy.

IMPACT ON FERTILITY

• Protects fertility.

IMPACT ON SEXUALITY

• May interfere with spontaneity.
• May make oral sex less enjoyable. (See caution on oral sex and AIDS, page 121.)
• Either partner may experience a warmth or burning sensation from foaming suppositories that may be perceived as unpleasant, although in some cultures the feeling of warmth is seen as a plus.

MOST SUCCESSFUL USERS

• Women who use consistently and correctly.
• Young women who do not want to use prescription methods.

WHO SHOULD NOT USE

• People with allergies to spermicides.
• Women who do not have good communication with partner(s) about sex.

• Couples in stable relationships have good continuation while continuation rates of single women who use spermicides as an occasional method vary widely.

COST FOR ONE YEAR

• $50

✳ FERTILITY AWARENESS ✳ ✳ ✳ ✳ ✳ ✳ ✳ ✳
(Natural Family Planning)

Over the last century, bits and pieces of information about hormones have emerged so that, today, ovulation can be readily detected in about 70 percent of women. In the late 1860s, Dr. Squire, a British physician, first observed that a precipitous rise in temperature roughly coincided with ovulation. In the 1930s, two Australian Catholic physicians, John and Evelyn Billings, researched and popularized the concept of "mucus observation" (also called "the ovulation method" or "the Billings method") as a scientific update to the old-fashioned and highly unreliable calendar rhythm method. As a result of the Billings' efforts, avoiding intercourse during the fertile time as a method of contraception became officially sanctioned by the Catholic Church. In the 1940s, physicians began recommending the use of basal body temperature (the lowest observable temperature each day) to help women who had difficulty getting pregnant to determine the optimum time for conception.

Today, observation of changes in cervical mucus, basal body temperature, and other bodily signs, has come to be known as "fertility awareness" or "natural family planning," and the concepts are used both for avoidance of pregnancy and as aids to conception.

Some people use natural family planning as their sole method of birth control, identifying the fertile time and keeping the penis out of the vagina (commonly referred to as "abstinence") for that interval. Others have adapted it to their own needs, using it quite successfully in combination with barrier methods.

Because of the period of abstinence required, effective natural family planning is ideally practiced with the cooperation of both partners, but some women who do not have steady partners also use it quite effectively. Even if you are young and inexperienced or have an unpredictable sex life, information about natural family planning can help you gain self-assurance, be more assertive about your contraceptive needs, minimize risk-taking, and lower your anxiety about getting pregnant.

How to Make Any Birth Control Method More Effective

Ovulation is initiated by the brain's hypothalamus, which stimulates the pituitary gland to signal the release of certain hormones, which in turn stimulate an egg to mature in the ovary. Each menstrual cycle and complex sequence of hormonal events results in the production of a mature egg which literally bursts through the wall of the ovary and begins its journey along the egg tube (fallopian tube) toward the uterus. If the egg is not fertilized within the first 24 hours it will begin to disintegrate. If it is fertilized, it will continue its sojourn along the tube and become implanted in the uterine wall in about a week.

Concurrently, another chain of events, also hormonally stimulated, is occurring. In the early part of the cycle, mucus-producing glands in the cervical canal secrete a thick, impenetrable, acidic mucus that is weblike in structure. This mucus, often called "infertile mucus," actually prevents sperm from entering the cervical canal. About day 10 or 11 of an average 28- to 30-day cycle, the mucus begins to change. The weblike structure modulates into parallel streams through which sperm can easily swim. The mucus becomes more fluid and alkaline, which nurtures the sperm and provides a hospitable environment in which they can live. If sperm are deposited near the unprotected cervix, it takes only about 15 seconds for them to dart up the open pathways within fertile mucus and into the cervical canal. The canal itself is a warren of crypts and alleyways in which the sperm can live, protected and nurtured by the fertile mucus. Gradually, over a four- or five-day period, the sperm leave the cervical canal, swimming up through the uterus and into the egg tubes.

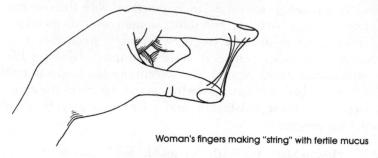

Woman's fingers making "string" with fertile mucus

For most women, the clear, viscous fertile mucus appears about day 11 or 12, and becomes progressively more profuse, peaking at midcycle—about day 14 or 15—then tapering off and ending about day 17 or 18. In the average 27- to 30-day cycle, ovulation usually occurs around midcycle or day 14 to 16, but it can sometimes occur earlier or later. Thus, there is a period of approximately eight days (or perhaps ten) when sperm can enter the cervical canal. These are the same eight to ten days in which an egg is released. For most women, ovulation appears to occur anywhere from 12 to 16 days before menstrual bleeding begins, regardless of whether they have an average, long, or short cycle.*

How to Identify Your Fertile Time

There are three commonly accepted signs of ovulation that any woman can readily identify:

The appearance of stretchy fertile mucus. Fertile mucus has distinctive characteristics that make it easy to identify. It has the color and consistency of egg white and will stretch between your fingers (see illustration on this page). Many women observe a distinct wetness or noticeable secretion coming from the vagina. Others notice the stretchy mucus on

---

* Barbara Kass-Annese, R.N., N.P., and Hal Danzer, M.D., *The Fertility Awareness Workbook* (Atlanta: Printed Matter, 1986).

toilet paper. Those who use a plastic speculum can look for a bubble or string of clear mucus coming out of the os. Ovulation is roughly coordinated with peak fertile mucus, but *you can get pregnant any time fertile mucus is present and you have unprotected intercourse.*

Changes in your basal body temperature. For many women, the basal body temperature drops slowly until about day 11 or 12 when estrogen production peaks and begins to drop and the production of progesterone begins to rise. Ovulation occurs about day 14 or 15. The heat-producing progesterone, which is produced in much higher quantities *after* ovulation, causes a noticeable rise in body temperature. Not all women have clear-cut temperature patterns, and those who do may not have them every cycle. For women who use fertility awareness as their sole method of birth control, it is only after a clear jump in temperature that it is safe to have unprotected intercourse. It is recommended that you use a basal body temperature thermometer, available at most drugstores, to chart your temperature changes.

Changes in the cervix. As ovulation approaches, the cervical os opens noticeably; the cervix itself may become puffy and soft and may move further back in the vagina. It is easiest to see the opening of the os by using a light, a mirror, and a plastic speculum.

In addition to fertile mucus, cervical changes, and basal body temperature, there are a number of other signs of ovulation that can often be noted, including fluid retention, an ovarian ache or pain (called "Mittleschmerz"), spotting, tender breasts, and changes in mood, energy level, libido, or tastes in food. For some women, these bodily signs are fairly clear-cut and predictable. For others, they may vary quite a bit from cycle to cycle.

There are several ways to learn more about how to identify your fertile time. Join a self-help group or a class at a women's clinic, family planning clinic, Catholic organization, or hospital. Some private teachers, who may advertise in alternative health publications, also conduct classes and discussion groups. While it is probably ideal to learn from an experienced teacher, there are several excellent books on fertility awareness that are generally available:

A Cooperative Method of Natural Birth Control
Margaret Nofziger
Summertown, Tenn.: The Book Publishing Company., 1978.

The Fertility Awareness Workbook
Barbara Kass-Annese and Hal Danzer
Atlanta: Printed Matter, 1986.

EFFECTIVENESS

• Theoretical Effectiveness 99%
• Highest Observed Effectiveness 80%–98%*
• Typical-User Effectiveness 85%*

HEALTH RISKS

• None.

HEALTH BENEFITS

• Heightened body awareness.

ADVANTAGES

• Use improves effectiveness of barrier methods.
• Offers opportunity for partner communication.
• Men can learn and participate.
• Develops self-esteem and self-reliance.
• Approved by Catholic Church.

DISADVANTAGES

• Requires an initial readjustment and commitment of time and energy for several months.
• Usually requires partner cooperation.
• Does not offer protection against sexually transmissible diseases.

IMPACT ON FERTILITY

• Does not protect fertility.

* Includes rhythm, basal body temperature and mucus observation.

- Offers opportunity to explore alternatives to intercourse during fertile time.
- Some people find having to keep the penis out of the vagina for seven to ten days each cycle inconvenient.
- Intercourse *after* ovulation can be spontaneous and free from anxiety about pregnancy.

MOST SUCCESSFUL USERS

- Committed couples who abide by the rules and who practice abstinence during the fertile time.
- Women who have high awareness of their bodies.

WHO SHOULD NOT USE

- Women or couples who are unwilling to commit the necessary time and effort to learn.
- Couples not willing to abstain from intercourse or use a barrier method during the fertile time.
- Women who are squeamish about touching their genitals or dealing with bodily secretions.
- Women who do not have the cooperation of their partners.

COST FOR ONE YEAR

- $5–$20 for basal body temperature thermometer.
- $0–$30 for books or literature.
- $0–$100 for classes.

✳ WITHDRAWAL ✳ ✳ ✳ ✳ ✳ ✳ ✳ ✳ ✳ ✳
(Coitus Interruptus)

Withdrawal is surely the cheapest, most convenient and risk-free method of birth control in the world. "It costs nothing, it cannot be forgotten when the couple goes away from home, the children cannot find it, the government cannot tax it, and it requires no medical supervision." * Ejaculation, in this simple technique, takes place outside of the vagina away from the

* Michael J. Free and Nancy Alexander, *Public Health Reports* (Sept.– Oct. 1976).

pubic area and inner thighs. Withdrawal is widely practiced in Europe today and has been used with excellent results in countries where birth control and abortion are prohibited. Young people frequently depend on this technique, because they often have sex at unexpected times or because they have not yet selected a method of birth control, although lack of experience or confidence may make it less effective.

In the United States, only about 2 percent of couples use withdrawal as their sole method of birth control, but many use it as a back-up or interim measure. Withdrawal is appropriately classified as a "male" method, but it does require co-operation of both partners to be effective. It does not work if the man cannot accurately control or predict his ejaculations.

Some couples don't mind the slight inconveniences that withdrawal imposes, and relish the freedom from pills, devices, and chemical goo. Having to anticipate ejaculation sometimes interferes with one or both partners' ability to achieve orgasm, especially the woman's, and some women object to having to focus more attention on the male orgasm than on their own. Some people actually enjoy the tension or suspense created by the anticipation of orgasm, at least on occasion, and manage to turn this disadvantage into a benefit.

Note *Withdrawal is far superior to no method at all.*

Although recent studies have not found sperm in the pre-ejaculatory fluid, it is commonly believed they can definitely be present in the pre-ejaculate for succeeding sessions of intercourse, unless the man has urinated. For repeated intercourse, the man should urinate and carefully wash his penis before insertion.

Dr. Christopher Tietze has proposed that while withdrawal is less effective than the Pill, IUD, condom, or diaphragm, it is theoretically "highly effective" and notes that this method is "mainly responsible for the early historical decline in birth rates among the peoples of northern and western Europe."

EFFECTIVENESS
• Theoretical Effectiveness 85%
• Use Effectiveness 76%–84%
• Typical-User Effectiveness 77%

HEALTH RISKS
• None.

HEALTH BENEFITS
• None.

ADVANTAGES
• Readily available.
• No apparatus.
• Nonprescription.
• Allows men to take responsibility for birth control.

DISADVANTAGES
• Not highly effective unless practiced in conjunction with fertility awareness.
• Requires some skill and commitment on the part of the man.

IMPACT ON FERTILITY
• Does not protect against sexually transmitted diseases, but theoretically the incidence of some conditions might be lower because semen is kept out of the vagina.

IMPACT ON SEXUALITY
• No interference from devices or spermicides.
• Not likely to cause injuries.
• Some couples find that withdrawal diminishes the enjoyment of the orgasmic phase of sexual response of one or both partners.

- Couples who use correctly and consistently.
- Men who have good control over ejaculation.
- People who want to avoid health risks or inconveniences associated with commercial birth control drugs or devices.

WHO SHOULD NOT USE

- Men who have difficulty anticipating and controlling ejaculation.

CONTINUATION RATE AFTER ONE YEAR

- Continuation rates are difficult to assess because so few people use as a sole method.

COST FOR ONE YEAR

- Nothing.

✳ ABORTION✳ ✳ ✳ ✳ ✳ ✳ ✳ ✳ ✳ ✳ ✳

Quite apart from blowing up clinics and terrorizing patients, the antiabortion movement can take credit for a more subtle and lasting kind of damage: It has succeeded in getting even pro-choice people to think of abortion as a "moral dilemma," an "agonizing decision" and related code phrases for something murky and compromising like the traffic in infant formula mix. In liberal circles, it has become unstylish to discuss abortion without using words like "complex," "painful," and the rest of the mealy-mouthed vocabulary of evasion. Regrets are also fashionable, and one otherwise feminist author writes recently of mourning, each year following her abortion, the putative birthday of her discarded fetus."†

Abortion techniques of the past included potions, insertion of various instruments into the uterus, crude surgical procedures and patently useless regimens such as wearing amulets and the performance of magical rites. Many of the

---

* In that it does not prevent conception, abortion is not technically a method of "contraception." It is, however, an important means of preventing birth (a concept that is actually older than conception prevention) and is included under the modern concept of "family planning."

† Barbara Ehrenreich, Hers Column, *New York Times*, Feb. 7, 1985.

techniques were exceedingly dangerous and frequently killed the woman as well as the fetus, causing the sixth-century Greek physician Soranos to decry their use and call for an emphasis on contraception.*

In 1869 when Pope Pius IX arbitrarily decreed that abortion was the moral equivalent to murder, pregnancy termination was in fact widely practiced by physicians and midwives, as well as by women themselves, who passed abortion techniques along from generation to generation like the family silver.

In the late 1970s, a virulent coalition of Catholic and Christian fundamentalist groups mounted an attack against abortion, openly aided and abetted by the Reagan administration and the media.† The heavily funded anti-abortion movement pulled out the big guns with *The Silent Scream,* a videotape purporting to show a nine-week fetus during an abortion. Although the inaccuracies of this film were effectively exposed by medical experts, the media had a field day and doubts were planted in the minds of many women.

In 1973, when the historic *Roe vs. Wade* and *Doe vs. Bolton* decisions were handed down by the U.S. Supreme Court, making pregnancy termination legal to twenty-four weeks, abortion-related deaths dropped by 40 percent. Today, "abortion is seven times safer than childbirth and carries approximately the same risk of death as a shot of penicillin, about one death in 100,000."‡

Dilation and curettage (D&C), euphemistically referred to as "dusting and cleaning" has been partially supplanted by the safer vacuum aspiration, a three- or four-minute procedure that could be done in a clinic or doctor's office under local anesthesia, or just as easily without, depending on the skill and touch of the practitioner. Vacuum aspiration is less

---

* Norman N. Himes, *The Medical History of Contraception* (New York: Schocken Books, 1970).

† A November 9, 1985 article, "Network Coverage of Abortion," in *TV Guide* documents the media's uncritical focus on the violence generated by anti-abortion groups.

‡ National Abortion Federation, "Twelve Years of Legal Abortion," 1985.

painful, has less risk of hemorrhage, more efficiently empties the uterus, is cheaper, and does not require general anesthesia.

In addition to vacuum aspiration and D&C, several other methods of abortion are used after the twelfth week of pregnancy. The dilation and evacuation (D&E) procedure, a modification of both the vacuum aspiration and the D&C, is generally done from thirteen to twenty weeks, but a few skilled practitioners in large urban areas will perform this procedure up to twenty-four weeks. The day before the D&E procedure, several sticks of compressed, dried seaweed called *laminaria* —about the size of kitchen matches—are inserted into the cervical canal. Overnight, the laminaria sticks absorb cervical secretions and expand, opening the cervix slowly and gently. The D&E procedure normally takes five to fifteen minutes, and women usually recover sufficiently to go home within an hour.

Use of the D&E is generally favored over the older *saline* abortion, in which a solution of sterile salt-water is injected into the uterus through the abdominal wall, killing the fetus and precipitating labor. Two other substances, *prostaglandins* and *urea*, either alone or in combination, are sometimes used to produce the same result as the *saline*. All of these procedures, called *instillations*, have a higher complication rate than the D&E and end with the delivery of a dead fetus, which can be far more traumatic for women than the D&E procedure. Instillation abortions often have to be supplemented with a D&C.

In 1979, Drs. Christopher Tietze and Sarah Lewit published the definitive study on the risk of death associated with the use of the major methods of birth control. They compared the risks of birth control to the risks of childbirth and of using abortion instead of birth control. The inescapable conclusion of this careful analysis is that *using a barrier method of birth control, backed up by early termination abortion in the case of an occasional failure, offers the lowest risk of death*—far lower than childbirth or the use of birth control pills or IUDs.*

* Christopher Tietze and Sarah Lewit, "Life Risks Associated with Reversible Methods of Fertility Regulation," *International Journal of Gynecological Obstetrics* 16 (1979), pp. 456–59.

Most women know if they want an abortion or not, without having to seek counseling. However, if you are ambivalent about the impact a birth or abortion may have on your life, talking it over with someone you trust could be very helpful.

Abortion services are listed in the Yellow Pages under "Abortion" and "Family Planning Services." Many clinics also advertise under "Health Services" in alternative and community newspapers. Certain Planned Parenthood clinics do abortions and all Planned Parenthood offices make referrals. Women's centers at universities are also good referral sources. The National Abortion Federation in Washington, D.C., which can be reached at (202) 546-9060, can give you the name of a clinic in your area that does abortions. Private-practice doctors often perform abortions, but usually prefer to do them under general anesthesia in a hospital—which can be risky and expensive, and is usually unnecessary. The best abortions are most often done at clinics which specialize in them.

EFFECTIVENESS

- 100%—Procedure must occasionally be repeated if all products of conception are not removed.

HEALTH RISKS

- Vacuum aspiration: 1 percent chance of infection or incomplete abortion.
- D&C: small chance of hemorrhage, blood clots, or incomplete abortion; small risk of death from anesthesia.
- D&E: Risks increase as pregnancy advances; infection, hemorrhage, blood clots, cervical laceration, uterine perforation; small risk of death from anesthesia.

HEALTH BENEFITS

- By having an abortion, you do not have to undergo the risks of pregnancy and childbirth.
- Significant mental health benefits for many women.

ADVANTAGES

- Safe: the earlier, the safer.
- Effective.

- Requires interaction with a physician.
- May be expensive for some women, especially teenagers.
- Temporary discomfort from procedure.
- Inconvenience of having to make arrangements for procedure and time for recovery.
- Some women may have difficulty explaining absence to parents, partners, employers.
- Short disruption of athletic activity.

IMPACT ON FERTILITY

- A post-abortion infection that is not treated promptly can cause pelvic inflammatory disease and possibly infertility.
- Contrary to popular belief, several suction abortions (without complications) will not affect fertility.

IMPACT ON SEXUALITY

- It is recommended that you forego intercourse for one to two weeks, or until post-abortion bleeding has stopped.

MOST SUCCESSFUL USERS

- Women or couples who do not have ambivalent feelings about abortion.

WHO SHOULD NOT USE

- Women or couples who are ambivalent about abortion.

COST FOR ONE YEAR

- $125–$1,500 per procedure; cost may vary from region to region, from clinic to doctor's office to hospital, and according to type of procedure; cost increases according to number of weeks of the gestation.

✳ MENSTRUAL EXTRACTION ✳ ✳ ✳ ✳ ✳ ✳

Before the legalization of abortion, women in California worked in underground abortion clinics and learned that the vacuum aspiration procedure was safe, simple, and easily adaptable to "home use." Based on illustrations in articles in Russian and Chinese medical journals, Lorraine Rothman, founder of the Orange County Feminist Women's Health Center in Santa Ana, California, developed a hand-operated apparatus similar in function and design to medical aspirators, but producing a gentler suction. Rothman and her colleagues at the Los Angeles Feminist Women's Health Center studied anatomy texts, learned sterile technique, and began extracting each other's periods on a regular basis. Later, women in Europe invented very serviceable mechanical aspirators of their own from used refrigerator motors. They found that extracting the period on or before the first day of a new cycle served several purposes: as a convenience, to shorten their periods and greatly reduce the menstrual flow; as a method of birth control; and to learn more about the menstrual cycle.* For fifteen years in various parts of the United States, England, Europe, Australia, and New Zealand and in Central and South America, lay women have practiced menstrual extraction with a remarkable safety record and have shared their knowledge with women in countries where abortion is illegal or where political conditions make giving birth an intolerable occurrence.

Although physicians and the general public often react in horror at the idea of lay women doing abortions on each other, they have, in fact, been doing them for thousands of years. The difference is that now they can do them safely and effectively using sterile technique and knowledge about the uterus and its functions.

In 1973, an international conference on menstrual extraction, or "menstrual regulation," attended by both professionals and lay practitioners, was held in Hawaii. A lively exchange of research and experiences occurred and the conference attendees concluded that menstrual extraction is "a helpful back-up when contraception fails," and that this con-

---

* The results of some of their studies appear in the Proceedings of the Menstrual Cycle Conference, 1979.

cept "is on the way to becoming an accepted gynecological procedure." *

✳ ALTERNATIVES TO PENIS-IN-VAGINA SEX ✳ ✳ ✳

In *The Hite Report*,† her groundbreaking study of women's sexuality, Shere Hite established that 70 percent of women do not achieve orgasm, or do not achieve it easily, through direct penis-vagina contact. Although orgasm is not always the goal in sexual activity, when it is it can be achieved for both partners in a variety of inventive and pleasurable—and for many women, more direct—ways without putting the penis into the vagina.

In addition to varying the sexual routine, couples practice alternatives to intercourse for various reasons: after injury or surgery or in advanced pregnancy, because of a physical disability, because one partner has a sexually transmitted disease like herpes or chronic trichomoniasis, or because the male has difficulty controlling ejaculation or difficulties with erection.

Some ideas for sexual innovation might be gleaned from books that include information on techniques used by lesbians and gay men in which vaginal penetration is not the focus of sexual activity, or books which cover sexual practices developed in other cultures, especially Tantric yoga, which emphasizes the sexual satisfaction of women.

EFFECTIVENESS

• Theoretical Effectiveness 99 + %
• Use Effectiveness: No studies have documented use.

HEALTH RISKS

• None.

---

* Theresa van der Vlugt and P. T. Piotrow, "Menstrual Regulation Update," *Population Reports*, Series F, no. 4, May 1974, p. 49.
† Shere Hite, *The Hite Report* (New York: Dell Publishing Co., 1976), p. 229.

HEALTH BENEFITS
• Excellent protection against sexually transmitted diseases.

ADVANTAGES
• Highly effective, free, always available.
• Offers an opportunity to share birth control responsibility.
• Does not require a prescription.
• Can be extremely erotic.
• Can serve to improve partner communication and mutual sexual enjoyment.
• Allows for sexual activity and orgasm when certain conditions may contraindicate penis-in-vagina sex.
• Can serve as an effective back-up or interim method.

DISADVANTAGES
• Penis *must* be kept out of the vagina to be effective.
• Requires good partner communication.

IMPACT ON FERTILITY
• Protects fertility.

IMPACT ON SEXUALITY
• Creates new ways to experience and enjoy sexual activity and improve communication.
• Can be enjoyed when one partner has an injury or physical disability.
• Can be used in later pregnancy as an interim, part-time, or back-up method.

MOST SUCCESSFUL USERS
• Couples who are not afraid to experiment.

WHO SHOULD NOT USE
• Anyone unwilling to follow the simple rule of keeping the penis out of the vagina should not use this method.

COST
• Nothing.

12 ✻ THE NEXT GENERATION:
Cervical Caps of the Future

If a man can write a better book, preach a better sermon or make a better mousetrap than his neighbors, though he build his house in the woods, the world will make a beaten path to his door.

—Ralph Waldo Emerson

The sixty-year-old Prentif is, without a doubt, the grande dame of existing cervical cap models. In spite of its inability to fit many women and its somewhat bulky design, it has endured because it is sturdy and serviceable. Although the Prentif is the only cap to be considered by the FDA for approval for distribution in the United States, it has two sister caps also manufactured by Lamberts, the Dumas and the Vimule, and two German cousins, the KaWe and the Contracon, both hard plastic models which are similar to ones which have been manufactured for many years by Milex-Western and Ortho in the United States.

More sophisticated cervical caps may be the wave of the future, offering a wide range of sizes, custom fitting, and both semi-permanent and disposable models. Very possibly, advances similar to those made in contact lenses will occur, both in terms of technology and in provision of services. Caps of the future may be made on the spot at extremely low cost and provided on a worldwide basis by trained paramedical technicians instead of by physicians. Given the bleak outlook for truly low-risk contraception, it is not hard to imagine that women, if not the world, will beat a pathway to the door of the resourceful researcher who designs a better cervical cap.

CURRENT MODELS

The Dumas

The Dumas cap, also referred to as the "vault" cap, is of French origin, and has been manufactured and distributed by Lamberts Ltd. for many years. This amber-colored, dome-shaped device looks like a diaphragm and comes in five sizes, from about 40 mm in its internal diameter to about 60 mm. Because it does not have a spring rim, the Dumas does not depend upon the protrusion of the pubic bone, as the diaphragm does, to stay in place. It fits directly over the cervix and stays in place, like the Prentif and other cervical caps, by suction and by burying its rim in the folds of musculature at the back of the vagina. Women who cannot be fit with the Prentif, and for that matter those who cannot use the diaphragm because the pubic bone is not prominent enough, may be able to use the Dumas without any trouble.

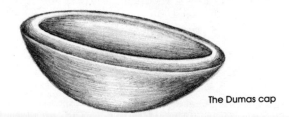

The Dumas cap

The best news since the approval of the Prentif is that Lamberts has expressed an intention to conduct the requisite animal studies on the Dumas and plans to submit the results to the FDA for approval sometime within the next two years. Perhaps in the meantime, many cap fitters will continue to provide the Dumas under Investigational Device Exemptions so that women who cannot use the Prentif will have another cervical cap option.

· Initially, practitioners in the United States did not exhibit much interest in the Dumas, but a few feminist clinics began to experiment with it and offered it when a woman could not use either the Prentif or the Vimule. The Washington Women's Self-Help group, the Atlanta Feminist Women's Health Center, and the Alternative Health Center of Seattle have fit many Dumas caps, and numerous other practitioners have provided them on a smaller scale.

Both caps stay on through a combination of suction and gripping, but, unlike the Prentif which settles directly onto the cervix, the Dumas envelops the cervix, covering it with its rounded dome, and buries its rim in the surrounding vaginal muscles.

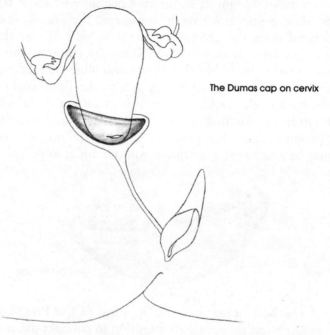

The Dumas cap on cervix

Karen Milgate, who has fit several hundred of the Dumas caps at Washington Women's Self-Help (WWSH), says that the Dumas seems to be particularly well suited for women who have cervixes that protrude less, which are irregular or softer after several births. "Women who have good vaginal muscle tone are the best candidates for the Dumas," she says. "If the vagina is very smooth, or the muscle tone is lax, I don't feel so secure about it. The only real contraindication that we've found is a very long cervix, but sometimes even then one of the larger sizes will work. . . . In checking fit, I use two fingers to feel for gaps on the part of the rim above the cervix, which is where they usually occur. I usually don't worry too much about the sections back and underneath. They are almost always secure," Milgate says.

Lynn Thogersen of the Atlanta Feminist Women's Health Center finds that it isn't so easy to predict who can or can't use the Dumas, but that "women with very fleshy vaginal walls seem to use it well." The combined Feminist Women's Health Centers study (including 5 clinics) fits about 300 Dumas caps a year and reports a use effectiveness rate of 97 percent.

Nurse Practitioner Linda Stein of the Alternative Health Center in Seattle reports that the effectiveness rates for the Dumas and the Prentif were nearly identical: 82.5 percent for the Dumas and 84.1 percent for the Prentif. This clinic also fits about 300 Dumas caps a year.

The Dumas cap was not included as a part of the Bernstein study, and was thus not eligible for approval along with the Prentif. Because this cap has not been widely studied, it is not known how many women might be able to use it, but it is clear that some women can use it with good results, and it could be a useful alternative for some of the women who cannot be fit with the Prentif. It might also be serviceable for some of the women whose partners have problems with the Prentif.

Perhaps the Dumas is the real solution to Dr. Edward Stim's dream of the "nonspermicide fit-free diaphragm," [*] in which "a small diaphragm . . . is held in place by the muscles high in the vaginal vault, with the soft rubber dome closely covering the cervix." This concept, which is well known but not taken very seriously in family-planning circles, is sometimes mentioned as a possible alternative to the "largest is best" philosophy of diaphragm fitting. Dr. Stim published his thoughtful, visionary article in 1980, but no one has ever tried to test his theory or duplicate his results. (For more information, see page 123.)

[*] Edward M. Stim, "The Nonspermicide Fit-free Diaphragm: A New Contraceptive Method," *Advances in Planned Parenthood* 15 (1980).

The Vimule

The amber-colored, bell-shaped Vimule is also of French origin and of the same vintage as the Prentif and the Dumas. Also manufactured by Lamberts, the Vimule comes in three sizes and has a flared rim that attaches itself to the vaginal walls surrounding the cervix as the Dumas does. Because it clings to the vaginal walls instead of to the cervix itself, this model does not require such a specific fit and can often be used by many of the women who cannot be fit with the Prentif. In fact, health workers at the Atlanta Feminist Women's Health Center have found that "the Vimule is sort of like a medium tee-shirt: almost any woman can wear one." Women whose partners experience discomfort from the rigid rim of the Prentif can often switch to the Vimule with good results. (See illustration of Vimule on page 29.)

Because of the controversy over the Vimule (described on page 28), it is not likely to be approved in the United States anytime soon. Dr. Koch has designed a Vimule without a rough edge, but his model remains untested.

Vimule proponents surmise that some of the women who got Vimules before the FDA prohibited importation are still using them without problems, and suggest that further follow-up on these cap users might offer some very useful data. And in spite of its problems in the United States, the Vimule is still manufactured by Lamberts, and can be ordered by individual practitioners or clinics in other countries.

The Test Cap

Spurred by renewed interest in the cervical cap and aware of the limitations of the Prentif, Lamberts attempted to design a new cap in 1981. This model, called simply the *test cap*, is made of the same amber-colored rubber as the Vimule and the Dumas, but of a much lighter weight and comes in six sizes, the inner diameter measuring from about 21 mm to 36 mm. This high-domed cap is quite similar in shape to Marie Stopes's long-time favorite, the Prorace cap, and bears a strong resemblance to the French pessary originally recommended by Emma Goldman and Margaret Sanger. Like the

Prentif, the test cap has a notch on its outer rim, but it does not have an inner suction ring. The apparent advantage of this model, aside from two additional sizes, is its lack of bulk. When in place, its minimal rim is far less likely to be felt by either a woman or her partner.

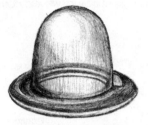

The test cap

When the test cap was first designed, Lamberts sent samples to many of its clients in the United States, but received surprisingly little interest. Some health workers in several feminist clinics tried them out on themselves, with mixed results. Some people thought the cap was too flimsy and did not hold the cervix firmly enough. "I tried one of the test caps myself," says Beverly Whipple, director of the Yakima Feminist Women's Health Center, "and found it quite comfortable and unobtrusive. And contrary to some people's predictions, it did not fall off." So far this cap has not been studied, so its true potential remains unclear.

German Caps

The most widely used cap manufactured in Europe is the German *KaWe* (pronounced "K.W.") cap. This hard clear plastic celluloid cap is manufactured by the Kirchner and Wilhelm company* in Stuttgart. A second German cap, the *Contracon* is made by Dr. Schweitzer, G.m.b.H., in Berlin. This milky-colored "Perlon" plastic cap comes in six sizes ranging from 22.5 mm to 33.5 mm.

A third European cap that is no longer manufactured is a conically shaped plastic cap that has a pinkish cast to it. Dr. Lehfeldt, who has one of these models in his "cervical cap museum," thinks that the conical shape may be superior to

* Heusteigstrasse 70, 700 Stuttgart 1, West Germany.

the hemispherical models because it has an ability to adjust to the shape of the cervix, especially as it expands during sexual activity. These plastic caps can be left in place during the entire intermenstrum.

COMPARISON OF A HEMISPHERICAL (KAWE) AND CONICAL CAP

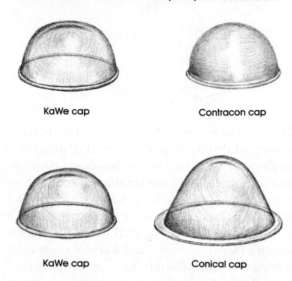

KaWe cap

Contracon cap

KaWe cap

Conical cap

U.S. Celluloid Caps

Both the KaWe and the Contracon are similar in appearance to two hard plastic caps manufactured in the United States by Ortho Pharmaceuticals and Milex-Western. According to Dr. Lehfeldt, both of these caps were prescribed by a few physicians for contraception, although the companies now contend that they were only intended to be used to hold sperm next to the cervix in artificial insemination. When the Pill came on the market in 1960, Ortho stopped making its cap and Dr. Lehfeldt bought up their entire stock so he could continue to provide them.

Milex still makes its cap today, but its only approved use is for artificial insemination. "We have heard that in the past, some doctors prescribed the device for other uses," says Mr. H. T. Milgrim, president of the small, family-owned company. Milgrim says that because of the threat of lawsuits,

Milex has no interest in trying to promote the caps for contraceptive purposes.

Ortho maintains the official fiction that it never manufactured a cervical cap, but the company appears to have a short memory. The company's plastic cap was one of the models used in the 1953 study done by Drs. Tietze, Lehfeldt, and Liebmann. A visit to the Museum of Contraception, established and maintained by Ortho's Canadian subsidiary, might clear up this official amnesia.*

In comparing the U.S.-manufactured plastic caps to the German-made *KaWe*, Dr. Koch observes, "The real difference is that the KaWe cap is more than a hemisphere—designed to stay on—while the Ortho and Milex models are less than a hemisphere—designed to fall off." This isn't a very good recommendation for either of these domestic models, but it is interesting to note that a cervical cap is presently manufactured in the United States, but that instead of being marketed as a contraceptive product, it is promoted for exactly the opposite reason: to promote conception by holding sperm against the cervix in artificial insemination.

Dr. Sein's Indian Cap

A photograph of a polyethylene plastic cervical cap appeared in a January 1976 *Population Reports* † on the global status of barrier methods. The report cites an unpublished paper entitled "Plastic Contraceptive Cervical Caps: An Ideal Contraceptive for Developing Countries," written in 1975 by Dr. Muang Sein, a New Delhi gynecologist. Dr. Sein's report is quoted as saying that "there have been no failures among 300 British and Indian women who were fitted with the device," but notes that follow-up was only for six months. The report also notes that "plans are now under way to mass produce the plastic cap." Apparently some limited trials using Sein's cap were conducted in England, but with inconclusive results.

* Museum of Contraception, Ortho Pharmaceuticals, Canada, 19 Green Belt Drive, Don Mills, Ontario, M3C 1L9, 416/449-9444.
† *Population Reports*, Series H, no. 4 (Jan. 1976).

FUTURE CAPS

Contracap

The *Contracap* looks like a large hemispheric soft contact lens and stays in place by surface tension—more like contact lenses than like cervical caps. The impetus for this intriguing line of investigation arose in 1974 through the collaborative efforts of dentist Robert Geopp and gynecologist Uwe Freese at the University of Chicago Medical Center. The two sought to design a custom-fit, spermicide-free cervical cap with a one-way valve for the release of secretions and menstrual fluid, that can be left in place for extended periods of time. Geopp and Freese applied the simple dental techniques for taking molds of the teeth and gums to making a mold of the cervix, in a process strikingly similar to that described by Dr. Wilde in 1838.

"We found that replicating the cervix was not that easy," says Geopp. "It is a mobile organ not backed up by bone. Even introducing a speculum often changes the shape of the musculature surrounding the cervix. You have to take a very passive impression to avoid distortions."

The two also experimented with a number of materials, both common and exotic, before they settled on Krayton, a

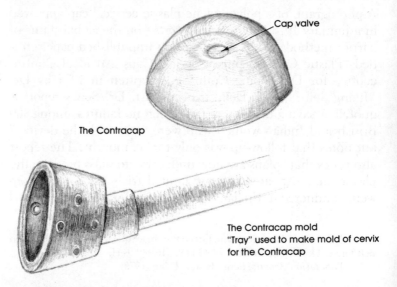

Cap valve

The Contracap

The Contracap mold
"Tray" used to make mold of cervix
for the Contracap

clear, pliable thermoplastic rubber developed by the Shell Chemical Company. They also worked very hard to develop a one-way valve which would allow secretions to seep out of the cap, but would not allow sperm to enter.

"The first valve was similar to a door," says Geopp. "Very viscous secretions could block it open. We modified it somewhat and it is now more like a valve-tunnel of varying lengths." The valve has presented certain design problems that have still not been satisfactorily solved.

Initial trials in both the United States and England yielded unacceptably high pregnancy rates, and the National Institutes of Health withdrew its financial support of the project after only six months in 1982. To date, there are few clues as to whether the Contracap failures are primarily due to dislodgements, lack of spermicide, use of tampons, the migration of sperm through the valve, or some combination of these factors.

A disappointing trial of the Contracap conducted at London's Royal Free Hospital yielded an unacceptably low effectiveness rate of 69 percent and the trial was canceled.* Walli Bounds, the midwife who coordinated the study, reports that in spite of the many pregnancies, nearly one third of the twenty-nine women in the study "found the cap highly acceptable and chose to continue its use beyond the closure of the trial."

Even though Contracap's one-way valve is not yet perfected, the technology for taking a cast of the cervix and making a custom-fit cap is amazingly simple—so simple, in fact, that impressions of the cervix can be taken and the caps constructed by trained paramedics.

In spite of Contracap's setbacks, this creative line of investigation may yet yield some useful results. Even in its present unperfected state, the Contracap improves over the traditional cap designs in several significant ways. Almost all women could be fit with such a cap. Because it can be safely

* Walli Bounds et al., "Clinical Trial of a Spermicide-free, Custom-fitted, Valved Cervical Cap (Contracap™)," *British Journal of Family Planning* 11, pp. 125–31.

left in place for extended periods, its use can be totally separated from sexual activity. It is not bulky and is unlikely to cause discomfort or injury to either the user or her partner and it should not interfere with sexual sensations.

No researcher should be criticized for thinking too big, but perhaps the goal of designing a cap with a complex outlet for secretions and intended to be kept in place for an entire year is too ambitious for the present. And many physicians will balk at placing *anything* on the cervix for more than a few days at a time. Why can't we, in the meantime, have custom-fit Contracaps, without valves, that women can place and remove at will?

In spite of the difficulties in perfecting this device, Dr. E. Ronald Atkinson, the current administrator of the Contracap project, has an optimistic outlook for the future. "New devices don't come into existence overnight," he maintains. "It takes an average of seven years from concept to implementation of any new product. So far, we feel we are progressing satisfactorily." Atkinson estimates that at this time, this custom device is only appropriate for about 15 percent of the general population, but refuses to see this relatively small number as a negative figure. If 35 million women need birth control at any one time, he points out, up to 5 million might be candidates for a custom-fit cervical cap.

Current German Research

While the resurgence of the Prentif has attracted much attention in the United States, a few West German researchers have been quietly investigating some of the basic problems of cap use and design, and experimenting with basic technology for making custom-fit caps simply and easily. Dr. Ingolf Schmid-Tannwald, who is on the faculty at Ludwig Maximilian University in Munich, directed the dissertations of two dental students who experimented with making negative molds of the cervix by infusing a silicon-based dental material around the cervix, using a speculum and a large syringe. These molds could then be used to make a custom-fit cervical cap. Schmid-Tannwald then reported on a small study he and two colleagues carried out in which molds were made of the cervixes of 40 women—the first step in the manufacture of a custom-fit cap.*

Ortho's "Diaphragm/Cap"

One promising new cap design that already appears to have bitten the dust is a spermicide-infused disposable "diaphragm" designed by Ortho Pharmaceuticals. Although the company calls it a "diaphragm," and apparently intended to market it as such, the device looks something like a styrofoam cervical cap, and might be more appropriately and honestly called a "dia-cap." This dia-cap, made from a lightweight porous plastic, is infused with nonoxynol-9 and, like the contraceptive sponge, is intended to be left in place for up to twenty-four hours and then discarded.

Ortho's insistence on calling the cap a "diaphragm" is curious, especially since it has no spring in its rim, looks like a cervical cap, and, in fact, stays on by suction. Since both the diaphragm and nonoxynol-9 are already approved by the FDA, approval would appear a certainty, with a minimum of testing, if acceptable effectiveness rates could be established. In 1985, several study sites were chosen and trials started, but the device was abruptly withdrawn from use, with vague references to "quality control" given as a reason.

Proctor & Gamble's "Double Cap"

In 1980, two Germans, J. L. Drobisch and T. W. Gongeon, designed a two-layered cap, which has a reservoir for spermicide. The inside layer is of silicon-polymer, a semi-permeable membrane which allows spermicide to seep out, and is covered by an outside layer of latex. Proctor & Gamble bought U.S. rights to the patent, but has not started any clinical trials so far.†

* I. Schmid-Tannwald, E. Graf, and W. Beitelschmidt, Individuelle Portioabdrücke beim Menschen. Erste klinische Ergebnisse. Mitteilungen der Gesellschaft fur praktische Sexualmedizin No. 4, May, 1984.
† Thomas Ludwig, *Zur Technik der Individuellen Abformung der Portio Vaginalis Uteri.* Inaugural-Dissertation zur Erlangung der Doktorwürde in der Zahnheilkunde an der Ludwig Maximilians-Universität zur München, 1983.

Dr. Koch's Ideal

Dr. James Koch is without a doubt the preeminent cervical cap researcher in the world. Soon after he began fitting Prentif caps in his practice, he became aware of its limitations and began thinking about ways to improve its basic design. He also undertook to design a cervical cap inserter/remover, but soon discovered this was no easy task. From the very beginning, Koch set out "to design a cap that will fit almost all women and be virtually foolproof—one that will be 99 percent effective and relatively hassle free." In early 1987, two of his designs were patented, and he applied for funding for clinical trials from the National Institutes of Health.

In the meantime, Dr. Bernstein is also gearing up to begin clinical trials on a slightly modified new model of the Prentif in Los Angeles.

Most people familiar with the state of the art regarding cervical caps admire the sturdy little Prentif and rejoice at its rediscovery, but would agree with Koch that "it isn't going to cut enough ice to serve the entire population." As Koch sees it, "approval of the Prentif should stimulate more funding and research into cervical caps, and that can't come too soon."

What does the future offer the millions of women in the United States and other countries currently experiencing the birth control crisis as a day-to-day reality? Realistically, they can probably expect the approval of the Dumas cap in the next two years. The new caps designed by Dr. Koch, and the one about to be tested by Dr. Bernstein, might, and perhaps a modified Vimule might, with good luck, see the light of day in five or six years. It remains to some energetic, well-funded researcher to push other caps, and their untested materials, through the necessary bureaucratic hurdles. Perhaps with an outburst of public interest in the Prentif, Ortho and Proctor & Gamble will put their designers to work to perfect this potentially useful model. And while the Contracap remains to be perfected, the dedicated research that has gone into its development should not be lost on researchers.

Given the bleak outlook for truly low-risk chemical contraception, more sophisticated cervical caps may well be the wave of the future, offering a wide range of sizes, custom fitting, and both semi-permanent and disposable models. Future caps may be provided on a worldwide basis by trained paramedical technicians casting and fitting caps on the spot, rather than by physicians. What about a custom-fit, feather-light plastic cap that could be worn for a week at a time after it is soaked for a few hours in a spermicidal solution? Such a cap might come with an inserter as handy and convenient as those used today for tampons and suppositories. Perhaps the Japanese will update the ancient bamboo-paper misugami, and market throwaway, spermicide-infused versions. Indeed, handy, disposable wax models might be fit by a woman herself with the help of a five-minute home-video cassette. Beeswax entrepreneurs take note.

None of these outlandishly simple suggestions is beyond the pale. We simply have to pay for their development.

The revival of the cervical cap has been a unique event in the history of modern contraception. Its impetus came not from the highly paid movers and shakers in the pharmaceutical industry or in public and private population control offices. It came from concerned feminist activists, health practitioners, and physicians who saw the limitations of high-technology birth control and whose priorities were and are focused on health and safety as well as effectiveness. Their dedication and unwavering faith in the cap has provided women with a significant new birth control option and has opened up intriguing possibilities in contraceptive research.

CERVICAL CAP INVESTIGATORS
1980–1987

ARKANSAS

Winslow Community Health
   Center
Janet L. Titus, M.D.
P.O. Box 270
Winslow, Ark. 72959
501/634-7071

ARIZONA

Arizona Family Health Center
Rob Cagen, N.D.
527 North Tucson Blvd.
Tucson, Ariz. 85791
602/795-8731

Biltmore Chiropractic
Elizabeth S. Ruman, D.C.
1444 W. Bethany Home Rd.
Phoenix, Ariz. 85013
602/957-4235

CALIFORNIA

Cidney Afriat, C.N.M.
966 Cass St., #200
Monterey, Calif. 93940
408/649-1144

Gerald Bernstein, M.D.
Women's Hospital

Los Angeles County/U.S.C.
   Medical Center
1240 N. Mission Rd.
Los Angeles, Calif. 90033

Judy Wittenberg Bravard, N.P.
12304 Santa Monica Blvd., #111
West Los Angeles, Calif. 90025
213/207-3705

Everywoman's Clinic
1936 Linda Dr.
Pleasant Hill, Calif. 94523
415/825-7900

Feminist Women's Health
   Center
330 Flume St.
Chico, Calif. 95926
916/891-1911

Health Care Center for Women
13320 Riverside Dr., #220
Sherman Oaks, Calif. 91423

International Women's Center
   for Planned Motherhood
Alan Gold, M.D.
6200 Wilshire Blvd., Suite 1008
Los Angeles, Calif. 90048
213/826-0871

Irwin Frankel, M.D.
George Weinberger, M.D.
2080 Century Park East, #1702
Los Angeles, Calif. 90067
213/277-1421 or 553-2777

Isla Vista Health Projects
Richard Ward, R.N.
970 Embarcadero Del Mar
Isla Vista, Calif. 993017
805/968-1511

Los Angeles Childbirth Center
Leslie Stewart, C.N.M.
575 Pier Ave.
Santa Monica, Calif. 90405
213/392-3931

Mendocino Coast Women's
    Center
P. Annie Mosher, C.N.M.
850 Sequoia Cir.
Fort Bragg, Calif. 95437
707/964-0259

Natural Childbirth Institute
Robin Ozerkis, C.N.M.
Nancy McNeese, C.N.M.
10862 Washington Blvd.
Culver City, Calif. 90230
213/559-6270

Oakland Feminist Women's
    Health Center
2930 McClure St.
Oakland, Calif. 94609
415/444-5676

Patricia O'Donnell, N.P.
6333 Wilshire Blvd., #101
Los Angeles, Calif. 90048
213/658-8224

Gayle Palmer, M.D.
1824 Hillhurst Ave.
Los Angeles, Calif. 90027
213/665-7835

Santa Cruz Women's Health
    Center
250 Locust St.
Santa Cruz, Calif. 95060
408/427-3500

Sherman Oaks Women's Health
    Center
Kolleen Squires, N.P.
4849 Van Nuys Blvd., #102
Sherman Oaks, Calif. 91403
213/784-0994

Grace Geyer Smith, M.D.
Student Health Service
University of California at
    Berkeley
Berkeley, Calif. 94720
415/643-8870

Gil Solomon, M.D.
18909 Sherman Way
Reseda, Calif. 91335
818/344-5141

South Bay Birth Alternative
Vicki Wolfrum-Cordesius,
    C.N.M.
264½ E. 22nd St.
San Pedro, Calif. 90731
213/832-4319

Westside Neighborhood Health
    Clinic
Margot Garcia, P.A.C.
628 Micheltorena
Santa Barbara, Calif. 93101
805/963-1546

Wholistic Health for Women
Suzann Gage
8235 Santa Monica Blvd., #201

West Hollywood, Calif. 90046
213/650-1508

Woman to Woman Health
Center
6950 Commerce Blvd.
Rohnert Park, Calif. 94928
707/792-1654

Woman to Woman Health
Center
Katy O'Leary and Elizabeth
Davis
1412 Cypress
Berkeley, Calif. 94703
415/525-9218 or 753-5997

Womancare
2850 6th Ave., Suite 311
San Diego, Calif. 92103
619/298-9352

Women's Choice Clinic
6221 Wilshire Blvd., #419
Los Angeles, Calif. 90048
213/938-9838

Women's Choice Clinic
2136 Market St
Redding, Calif. 96002
916/243-4680

Women's Choice Clinic
1200 Sonoma Ave.
Santa Rosa, Calif. 95405
707/575-8212

Women's Need Center
Martha B. Fox
1698 Haight St.
San Francisco, Calif. 94117
415/221-7371

COLORADO

Boulder Valley Clinic
Kathleen Podboy

2346 Broadway
Boulder, Colo. 80302
303/442-1694

Fort Collins Women's Clinic
Kelvin F. Kesler, M.D.
Carol Krakauer
1120 E. Elizabeth, Building F
Fort Collins, Colo. 80521
303/493-7442

Margaret Norton, R.N.P
1755 Gilpin St.
Denver, Colo. 80218
303/399-4122

Women's Health Service Clinic
111 E. Dale St.
Colorado Springs, Colo. 80903
303/471-9492

CONNECTICUT

Barbara Rassow, D.C.
772 Post Road East
Westport, Conn. 06880
203/226-7722

Women's Health Services
Evelyn C. Kieltyka
314 Prospect St.
New Haven, Conn. 06511
203/777-4781

Yale Nurse-Midwifery Practice
855 Howard Ave.
New Haven, Conn. 06510
203/785-2423

FLORIDA

The Tallahassee Birth Center
260 E. 6th Ave.
Tallahassee, Fla. 32303
904/224-0490

Gainesville Women's Health
Center

FLORIDA (*continued*)

Max Suter, M.D.
805 S.W. 4th Ave.
Gainesville, Fla. 32601
904/377-5055

GEORGIA

Feminist Women's Health Center
580 14th St., N.W.
Atlanta, Ga. 30318
404/874-7551

ILLINOIS

Suzanne Trupin, M.D.
301 East Springfield Ave.
Champaign, Ill. 61820
217/356-3736

IOWA

Emma Goldman Clinic for Women
227 North Dubuque St.
Iowa City, Iowa 52240
319/337-2111

MARYLAND

Hillcrest Clinic
Horace Ward, Jr., M.D.
5602 Baltimore National Pike, #600
Baltimore, Md. 21228
301/788-4400

MASSACHUSETTS

Berkshire Ob-Gyn Associates
Michael J. Shreefter, M.D.
510 North St.
Pittsfield, Mass. 01201
413/499-4161

Hampshire Obstetrical & Gynecological Associates
Phyllis Smith, R.N.
264 Elm St.
Northampton, Mass. 01060
413/584-2303

James Koch, M.D.
1037 Beacon St.
Brookline, Mass. 02146
617/277-0700

MICHIGAN

Primary Care Nursing Group
Patricia Natale, R.N.
4201 St. Antoine
Detroit, Mich. 48201
313/745-4774

MINNESOTA

Duluth Community Health Center
Jan Gerber, B.S.N.
2 E. 5th St.
Duluth, Minn. 55805
218/724-1497

Women's Health Care Associates
Deborah Boehm, N.P.
1203 Lagoon Ave. South
Minneapolis, Minn. 55408
612/827-5501

MONTANA

Blue Mountain Women's Clinic
B. J. Bauermeister, N.P.
Douglas Webber, M.D.
715 Kensington, Suite 24
Missoula, Mont. 59801
406/721-1646

Mikelann Caywood–Baerg, C.N.M.
116 South Q St.
Livingston, Mont. 59407
406/222-0084

NEW HAMPSHIRE

Brian Beattie, M.D.
Box 32, North Rd.
Lancaster, N.H. 03584
603/788-2521

Concord Feminist Health Center
38 S. Main Street
Concord, N.H. 03301
603/225-2739
Rodney Feldgate, M.D.
Lin-Wood Medical Center
Lincoln, N.H. 03251
603/745-8103

Portsmouth Feminist Health Center
232 Court St.
Portsmouth, N.H. 03801
603/436-7588

Women's Health Care Associates of Concord
33 Warren St.
Concord, N.H. 03301
603/228-0134

NEW MEXICO

Women's Health Services
Saundra K. McKenna, C.N.M.
839 Paseo de Peralta, #D
Santa Fe, N.M. 87501
505/988-8869

NEW YORK

Niels H. Lauersen, M.D.
784 Park Ave.
New York, N.Y. 10021
212/744-4222

Hans Lehfeldt, M.D.
110 E. 82nd St.
New York, N.Y. 10028
212/517-8185

Ronnie Lichtman, C.N.M.
Susan Papera, C.N.M.
12 W. 72nd St.
New York, N.Y. 10023
212/724-5974

University of Rochester School of Nursing
Mary Sprik, R.N.
Leslie Skillman, R.N.
601 Elmwood Ave.
Rochester, N.Y. 14620
716/275-2375

Womancap
115 E. 23rd St., 2nd Floor
New York, N.Y. 10010
212/529-8489

Women's Care
Richard Lumiere, M.D.
235 E. 67th St.
New York, N.Y. 10022
212/734-5700

NORTH CAROLINA

University of North Carolina at Chapel Hill
Student Health Service
Peggy Norton, N.P.
Chapel Hill, N.C. 27541
919/966-2281

OHIO

Community Family Health Center
Nancy Perkins, C.N.M.
Peter Harrison, M.D.
1043 E. Weber Rd.
Columbus, Ohio 43211
614/268-7531

OKLAHOMA

Charles D. Taylor, M.D.
1117 North Shartel, #200

Oklahoma City, Okla. 73103
405/232-9561

OREGON

Feminist Women's Health
Center
6510 S.E. Foster Rd.
Portland, Oreg. 97206
503/777-7044

Health Practitioner Clinic
Bette Seagren, N.P.
923 S.W. 4th St.
Canby, Oreg. 97013
503/263-6611

Paul Kaplan, M.D.
Jeannie Merrick, N.P.
Gynecology and Infertility
677 E. 12th Ave, Suite 470
Eugene, Oreg. 97401
503/683-1559

Bonnie Malone, D.C.
385 Main St.
Sisters, Oreg. 97759
503/549-7141

Nurse Practitioner Clinic
Beryl Cook, R.N.
15 N. Morris St.
Portland, Oreg. 97229
503/667-8127

Siuslaw Rural Health Center
Meadow Martell
Box 12326, Tide Route
Swisshome, Oreg. 97480
503/268-4433

Women's Clinic and Birth
Center
Lisa Mae Leek, C.N.M.
3388 Merlin Rd.

Grants Pass, Oreg. 97526
503/474-5566

PENNSYLVANIA

Elizabeth Blackwell Health
Center for Women
1124 Walnut St.
Philadelphia, Pa. 119107
215/923-7577

RHODE ISLAND

Rhode Island Women's Health
Collective
50 Rounds Ave.
Providence, R.I. 02907
401/461-0280

TENNESSEE

Knoxville Center for
Reproductive Health
Robert Mueller, M.D.
1547 W. Clinch Ave.
Knoxville, Tenn. 37916
615/637-3816

UTAH

Utah Women's Clinic
Grant P. Bagley, M.D.
515 S. 400 East
Salt Lake City, Utah 84111
801/531-9192

VERMONT

Vermont Women's Health
Center
336 North Ave.
Burlington, Vt. 05401
802/863-1386

VIRGINIA

Northern Virginia Women's
Medical Center

Study Results from the Cervical Cap Investigators

The following chart contains information obtained from more than 90 study sites—nearly all of the Cervical Cap Investigators—that provided caps both before and during FDA regulation. Since the FDA did not require data to be submitted in any particular format, the methodologies, standards, and scope of the studies and follow-up rates varied widely, it is not possible to draw any hard conclusions from this data. It is possible, however, to detect some trends regarding fitting rates, sizes most frequently fit, spermicide use, and the length of time women keep the cap in place. The chart also provides a rough estimate of how many women have participated in cervical cap research since 1977.

Practitioners figured effectiveness rates according to the Life Table method or the Pearl Index (see page 106 for information on these two methodologies) or by performing a simple mathematical computation. Even though the translation may not be exact, for purposes of consistency all figures have been expressed in terms of effectiveness rather than in terms of failure.

Key to Effectiveness Rates:

T = Theoretical effectiveness for women who said that they used their caps correctly and consistently for every session of intercourse

u = Use effectiveness rate for women who may not have used their caps consistently

c = Combined theoretical and use effectiveness rates

Note:

● Published studies have been marked with an (*).

● Effectiveness rates are given only for the Prentif cavity rim cervical cap.

● Some figures have been estimated.

	EFFECTIVE-NESS RATE	METHOD OF ANALY-SIS	NUMBER OF STUDY SITES	NUMBER OF WOMEN REPORTED ON	TOTAL NUMBER OF WOMEN FIT	PERCENT OF WOMEN FIT	SIZES MOST FREQUENTLY FIT	PERCENT OF WOMEN USING SPERMI-CIDE	GENERAL LENGTH OF CAP WEAR	TYPES OF CAPS FIT
Cydney Afriat, C.N.M. Monterey, Calif.	100% T 90% U	%	1	20	20	90%	25 mm	100%	24 hrs.	Prentif

Clinic										
Alternative Health Center, Linda Stein, N.P., Seattle, Wash.	91% T / 84% U	%	1	892	892	99%	22 mm / 25 mm	66%	8 hrs.–7 days	Prentif, Dumas
*Gerald Bernstein, M.D., Los Angeles, Calif.	96% T / 82% U	Life Table	8	581	581	33%	22 mm / 25 mm	100%	36 hrs.	Prentif
Elizabeth Blackwell Health Center, Philadelphia, PA.	91% C	Life Table	1	704	1,000	70%	22 mm / 25 mm	94%	24 hrs.–7 days	Prentif, Vimule
Bread & Roses Women's Health Center, Milwaukee, Wis.	97% C	Life Table	1	823	1,500	95%	25 mm	97%	72 hrs.–7 days	Prentif, Vimule
Blue Mountain Women's Clinic, Missoula, Mont.	98% T / 96% U	%	1	56	144	100%	25 mm	100%	72 hrs.	Prentif
Michaelann Caywood-Baerg, Livingston, Mont.	100% T / 97% U	%	1	40	40	100%	25 mm	100%	72 hrs.	Prentif
Chelsea Women's Health Team, New York, N.Y.	90% C	Fearl Index	1	329	2,500	80%	22 mm / 25 mm	89%	8–72 hrs.	Prentif, Vimule
Community Family Health Center, Peter Howison, M.D., Columbus, Ohio	—	—	1	150	—	99%	22 mm	100%	72 hrs.	Prentif
*Johan Eliot, M.D., Ann Arbor, Mich.	82% C	—	8	1,025	2,200	40–50%	22 mm / 25 mm	80%	72 hrs.	Prentif, Vimule
Emma Goldman Clinic for Women, Iowa City, Iowa	97% T / 89% U	Life Table	4	1,103	1,103	76%	25 mm / 28 mm	97%	6–48 hrs.	Prentif, Dumas, Vimule
Federation of Feminist Women's Health Centers, Atlanta, Ga./Los Angeles, Calif.	98% T / 97% U	%	8	2,445	3,000	80%	28 mm	49%	24–48 hrs.	Prentif, Dumas, Vimule
Feminist Women's Health Center, Portland, Oreg.	97% T / 88% U	%	1	231	800	N/A	25 mm / 28 mm	75%	24–72 hrs.	Prentif, Dumas, Vimule

	EFFECTIVENESS RATE	METHOD OF ANALYSIS	NUMBER OF STUDY SITES	NUMBER OF WOMEN REPORTED ON	TOTAL NUMBER OF WOMEN FIT	PERCENT OF WOMEN FIT	SIZES MOST FREQUENTLY FIT	PERCENT OF WOMEN USING SPERMICIDE	GENERAL LENGTH OF CAP WEAR	TYPES OF CAPS FIT
Fort Collins Women's Clinic Fort Collins, Colo.	98% T 96% U	%	1	46	46	97%	22 mm	100%	8 hrs.	Prentif
Hampshire Ob-Gyn Association Northampton, Mass.										
Health Practitioner Clinic Bette Gay Seagren, N.P. Canby, Oreg.	90% T	%	1	290	290	70%	22 mm 25 mm	N/A	24 hrs.	Prentif
Hillcrest Clinic Baltimore, Md.	98% C	%	1	65	65	—	—	—	—	Prentif
*James P. Koch, M.D. Brookline, Mass.	91.6% C	Life Table	1	371	3,500	50%	22 mm	67%	3–7 days	Prentif
Knoxville Center for Reproductive Health Knoxville, Tenn.	91% T 83% U	%	1	496	496	88%	22 mm 25 mm	80%	24–48 hrs.	Prentif
*Niels H. Lauersen, M.D. New York, N.Y.	77% C	Pearl Index	1	217	—	—	—	91%	—	Prentif
*Hans Lehfeldt, M.D. Irving Sivin, M.D. New York, N.Y.	88% T 81% U	Pearl Index	1	130	—	85%	22 mm 25 mm	—	—	Prentif
Los Angeles Cervical Cap Study Los Angeles, Calif.	89% C	Life Table	14	361	3,000	75%	N/A	80%	1–4 days	Prentif
Mendocino Coast Women's Health Center Fort Bragg, Calif.	67% T 56% U	%	1	42	42	88%	25 mm 28 mm	100%	1–3 days	Prentif Vimule

Provider / Location										
Jeannie Merrick, N.P. Eugene, Oreg.	98% T 87% U	%	1	81	81	99%	25 mm 28 mm	99%	N/A	Prentif
Mount Baker Planned Parenthood Bellingham, Wash.	97% T 92% U	%	1	98	98	63%	22 mm 25 mm	N/A	N/A	Prentif
New Hampshire Feminist Health Center Concord and Portsmouth, N.H.	92% C	%	4	880	880	67%	22 mm 25 mm	97%	72 hrs.	Prentif
Northern Virginia Women's Medical Center Alexandria, Va.	91% C	Pearl Index	1	54	54	93%	25 mm 28 mm	95%	8–72 hrs.	Prentif
Oakland Feminist Women's Health Center Oakland, Calif.	91% C	%	8	4	780	—	25 mm 28 mm	80%	8–72 hrs.	Prentif Dumas Vimule
Santa Cruz Women's Health Center Santa Cruz, Calif.	86% C	%	1	775	775	77%	22 mm 25 mm	99%	N/A	Prentif Dumas
Mimi Secor, N.P. Cambridge, Mass.	96% T 92% U	%	1	500	500	70%	25 mm 28 mm	N/A	N/A	Prentif
Charles D. Taylor, M.D. Oklahoma City, Okla.	90% C	%	1	35	35	98%	22 mm 25 mm	N/A	N/A	Prentif
Jaret Titus, M.D. Winslow, Ark.	85% T 80% U	Life Table	1	57	57	83%	22 mm	90%	36–72 hrs.	Prentif
Suzanne Trupin, M.D. Champaign, Ill.	82% C	Life Table	1	149	149	90%	22 mm 25 mm	N/A	3–10 days	Prentif
University of Rochester School of Medicine Mary Sprik, R.N. Rochester, N.Y.	95% T 84% U	Life Table	1	117	280	93%	25 mm 28 mm	N/A	36–72 hrs.	Prentif
Utah Women's Health Center Salt Lake City, Utah	92% C	%	1	217	1,000	95%	22 mm	99%	24–72 hrs.	Prentif

	EFFECTIVE-NESS RATE	METHOD OF ANALY-SIS	NUMBER OF STUDY SITES	NUMBER OF WOMEN REPORTED ON	TOTAL NUMBER OF WOMEN FIT	PERCENT OF WOMEN FIT	SIZES MOST FREQUENTLY FIT	PERCENT OF WOMEN USING SPERMI-CIDE	GENERAL LENGTH OF CAP WEAR	TYPES OF CAPS FIT
Vermont Women's Health Center Burlington, Vt.	83% C	%	3	269	269	37%	22 mm	99%	6–72 hrs.	Prentif Dumas Vimule
Washington Women's Self-Help Washington, D.C.	95% C	%	1	1,268	1,650	75%	25 mm	78%	24–48 hrs.	Prentif Dumas Vimule
Westside Neighborhood Medical Clinic Santa Barbara, Calif.	—	N/A	1	102	102	—	25 mm	100%	10–72 hrs.	Prentif
Woman to Woman San Francisco, Calif.	91% T 91% U	%	1	112	112	98%	25 mm	70%	6–72 hrs.	Prentif Dumas
*Women's Health Care Associates Minneapolis, Minn.	81% T	Pearl Index	1	76	76	N/A	22 mm 25 mm	N/A	8–72 hrs.	Prentif
Women's Health Services Clinic Colorado, Springs, Colo.	—	%	1	910	910	80%	22 mm 25 mm 28 mm	99%	10–72 hrs.	Prentif
Women's Health Services New Haven, Conn.	92% C	%	1	40	181	67%	22 mm	100%	8–24 hrs.	Prentif
Women's Needs Center San Francisco, Calif.	89% T	Pearl Index	1	74	280	50%	22 mm	99%	10–72 hrs.	Prentif
Yakima Feminist Women's Health Center Yakima, Wash.	95% T 93% U	%	1	301	1,795	90%	22 mm 25 mm	55%	12–48 hrs.	Prentif Dumas Vimule

BIBLIOGRAPHY

Allbutt, Henry Arthur. *The Wife's Handbook*. 3d ed. London: J. W. Ramsey, 1886.

American Journal of Public Health 71 (2), Feb. 1981. "APHA Policy Statements 8003: Cervical Cap." Resolution sponsored by the Women's Caucus. Passed by the governing body.

"Another Barrier to Pregnancy." *Time*, Jan. 26, 1981.

Arthur, Carol. "Customized Cervical Cap: Evolution of an Idea." *Journal of Nurse-Midwifery* 25 (6), Nov.–Dec. 1980.

Bernstein, Gerald S. "Final Report: Use-Effectiveness Study of Cervical Caps. July 1, 1981–Mar. 31, 1986." Contract No. N01-HD-1-2804, Contraceptive Development Branch, Center for Population Research, National Institute of Child Health and Human Development, National Institutes of Health, Bethesda, Md. 20892.

———. "The Los Angeles Multicenter Study of the Cervical Cap." Proceedings: Canadian Committee for Fertility Research. Conference held at Hotel La Sapinière, Val David, Quebec, Canada, Nov. 24–25, 1983.

———, Linda H. Kilzer, Anne H. Coulson, Robert M. Nakamura, Grace G. Smith, Ruth Bernstein, Ron Frezieres, Virginia A. Clark and Carl Coan. "Studies of Cervical Caps I. Vaginal Lesions Associated with Use of the Vimule Cap." *Contraception* 26 (5), Nov. 1982.

Blowney, Janey. "Cervical Caps: An Old Device Finds New Favor." *Brigham and Women's Hospital News*, Winter 1981.

Boehm, Deborah. "The Cervical Cap: Effectiveness as a Contraceptive." *Journal of Nurse-Midwifery* 28 (1), Jan.–Feb. 1983.

Boston Women's Health Book Collective. *The NEW Our Bodies, Ourselves*. New York: Simon & Schuster, 1984.

Bounds, Walli, Ali Kubba, Yunus Tayob, Angela Mills and John Guillebaud. "Clinical Trial of a Spermicide-free, Custom-fitted,

Valved Cervical Cap (Contracap™)." *British Journal of Family Planning* 11, 1986.

Brillman, Judith. "The Cervical Cap." 1979. Article written for and distributed by the Boston Women's Health Book Collective.

Canavan, Patricia Ann and Claudia Ann Lewis. "The Cervical Cap: An Alternative Contraceptive." *Journal of Obstetrics and Gynecology Nursing* 10 (4), July–Aug. 1981.

"Cervical Cap May Have FDA Market Approval by Spring of 1987." *Contraceptive Technology Update*, Aug. 1986.

"Cervical Cap Stirs Interest of Practitioners and Patients." *Contraceptive Technology Update*, Dec. 1980.

"Cervical Cap Study Finds 8% Failure Rate; Users Highly Educated." *Family Planning Perspectives* 18 (1), Jan.–Feb. 1986.

"Cervical Caps, Diaphragms Provide Equal Protection from Pregnancy." *Contraceptive Technology Update*, Mar. 1986.

"Cervical Cap's Effectiveness Hampered by Dislodgement, Rubber Erosion." *Family Planning Perspectives* 18 (5), Sept.–Oct. 1986.

Chalker, Rebecca. "Cervical Cap Update." *Glamour*, Mar. 1983.

———. "New-Choice Birth Control: 'The Cap.' " *Self*, Dec. 1983.

Cherniak, Donna. *A Book About Birth Control*. 3d ed. Montreal: The Montreal Health Press, 1984.

Connell, Elizabeth B. "Cervical Caps." *Medical Aspects of Human Sexuality*, Mar. 1978.

"Contracap Makes Crucial Changes for Expanded Trials." *Contraceptive Technology Update*, Oct. 1983.

Cruikshank, Barbara. "Multicentered Study of Cervical Cap." Seminar on Current and Future Fertility Research, Quebec, Canada, 1982.

Culverwell, Melissa. "Is There a Cervical Cap in Your Future?" *Medical Self Care*, Summer 1983.

"Current Cervical Caps Often Fail to Meet Expectations." *Ob-Gyn News* 16 (1), Jan. 1, 1981.

Curtin, Janet. "The Cervical Cap: What Next?" *Womanwise*, New Hampshire Feminist Health Center, Summer 1985.

"Customized Cervical Caps May Offer Women a New, Non-Invasive Birth Control Method." University of Chicago and Pritzker School of Medicine, *Reports* 27 (2), Spring 1979.

Denniston, George C. and D. Putney. "The Cavity Rim Cervical Cap." *Advances in Planned Parenthood* 16, 1981.

Dickinson, Robert Latou. *Control of Conception*. Baltimore: The Williams & Wilkins Co., 1938.

———— and W. E. Morris. *Techniques of Conception Control*. Baltimore: The Williams & Wilkins Co., 1949.

Dillon, Sheila. "Birth Control: The New Findings." *McCalls*, Apr. 1981.

Downey, Alice. "Cervical Cap Update: HEW Discovers the Cervical Cap." *Womanwise* (New Hampshire Feminist Health Center), Winter 1979.

————. "Cervical Cap Brigade Converges on Lebanon." *Womanwise* (New Hampshire Feminist Health Center), Winter–Spring 1979.

————. "Cervical Cap Workshop Held." *Womanwise* (New Hampshire Feminist Health Center), Summer 1978.

Drobisch, J. L., and T. W. Gongeon. "Europischer Patentschrift für Proctor & Gamble." no. 0009517, Apr. 16, 1980.

Drohojowska, Hunter. "Alternative Birth Control: The Fight for Cervical Caps." *L. A. Weekly*, Jan. 30, 1980.

Eliot, Johan, Leslie Anderson and Stan Bernstein. "Progress Report on a Study of the Cervical Cap." *Journal of Reproductive Medicine* 30 (10), Oct. 1985.

Fairbanks, Betsy and Beth Scharfman. "The Cervical Cap: Past and Current Experience." *Women & Health* 5 (3), Fall 1980.

Finch, B. E. and H. Green. "Balls, Feathers and Caps." In *Contraception Through the Ages*. Springfield, Ill.: Charles C. Thomas, 1963.

Findlay, Steve. "Private, Public Groups in Pitched Battle Over Cervical Cap Use." *Ob-Gyn News*, Oct. 1, 1980.

Fischer-Duckelmann, A. *Die Frau als Hausartzin*. Stuttgart: Suddeutsches Verlags-Institut, 1905.

Foote, E. B. "A Step Backward." New York: Murray Hill Publishing Co., 1975.

Galen, Michele. "Birth-Control Options Limited by Litigation." *The National Law Journal*, Oct. 20, 1986.

Gallagher, Dana M. "The Cervical Cap: Issues in the Food and Drug Administration's Regulatory Approval System." Unpublished Thesis, UCLA School of Public Health, June 1986.

Gentile, Gwen P. and Donald W. Helbig. "Barrier Contraceptives and Spermicide: Revealed Wisdom Reconsidered." Paper presented to the Association of Planned Parenthood Physicians, Denver, Colorado, Oct. 4, 1980.

Geopp, Robert and Uwe Freese. "A Fitted Cervical Cap." *Medical News International Report* 4, Mar. 31, 1980.

Gollub, Erica, "Test Case for U.S. Regulatory Politics." *Health PAC Bulletin*, Sept. 1986.

————. "Use of the Cervical Cap Among a Clinic Population: Aspects of Acceptability and Effectiveness." Unpublished, 1984.

Gordon, Linda. *Woman's Body, Woman's Right: A Social History of Birth Control in America*. New York: Penguin, 1977.

Grafenberg, Ernest and Robert L. Dickinson. "Conception Control by Plastic Cervix Cap." *Western Journal of Surgery, Obstetrics and Gynecology* 52 (8), Aug. 1944.

Hatcher, Robert A., Felicia Guest, Felicia Stewart, Gary K. Stewart, James Trussell, Sylvia Cerel and Willard Cates. *Contraceptive Technology 1986–1987*. New York: Irvington Publishers, 1986.

Himes, Norman E. *Medical History of Contraception*. New York: Schocken, 1970.

"Imported Cervical Caps Have FDA's Temporary Blessing." *Medical World News*, Nov. 24, 1980.

Jackson, Marianne, Gary S. Berger and Louis G. Keith. *Vaginal Contraception*. Boston: G. K. Hall, 1981.

Johnson, Joann M. "The Cervical Cap: A Retrospective Study of an Alternative Contraceptive Technique." *American Journal of Obstetrics and Gynecology* 148 (5), Mar. 1, 1984.

Johnson, Mary Alice. "The Cervical Cap as a Contraceptive Alternative." *Nurse Practitioner* 10 (1), Jan. 1985.

Kabanova, A. "Mechanical Methods of Contraception." *Journal of Contraception* 1 (3), 1936.

Kafka, K. "Die Adhesions-Modellkappe." *Wiener Medizinische Wochenschrift* 22, 1908.

————. "Über den Neuen Kappenverschluss des Muttermundes und Seine Indikation." *Klinisch-Therapeutische Wochenschrift* 50, 1908.

————. "Über Kappenbehandlung." *Wiener Medizinische Wochenschrift* 41, 1908.

Katchadorian, H. A. and Donald T. Lunde. *Fundamentals of Human Sexuality*. New York: Henry Holt & Co., 1972.

Katchian, A. "Coil Chemistry and Cervical Cap." *The Lancet*, Mar. 26, 1972.

Kennedy, D. M. *Birth Control in America: The Career of Margaret Sanger*. New Haven: Yale University Press, 1970.

King, Liz. *The Cervical Cap Handbook for Users & Fitters*. The Emma Goldman Clinic for Women, 227 North Dubuque, Iowa City, Iowa 52240, 1981.

Kintzing, J. M. "Cervical Cap." *Mademoiselle*, Aug. 1980.

Koch, James. "The Prentif Contraceptive Cervical Cap: Acceptability Aspects and Their Implications for Future Cap Design." *Contraception* 25 (2), Feb. 1982.

———. "The Prentif Contraceptive Cervical Cap: A Contemporary Study of Its Clinical Safety and Effectiveness." *Contraception* 25 (2), Feb. 1982.

Konikow, Antoinette F. *Physicians' Manual of Birth Control*. New York: Buchholz, 1931.

———. "Report on Experience with the French Pessary." New York: *The Birth Control Review*, 1921. Proceedings of the First American Birth Control Conference. Nov. 11–13, New York City, 1921.

Lauersen, Niels H., Kathleen H. Wilson, Zoe R. Graves, Ford Calhoun, Lori E. Leeds and Yanni Antonopoulos. "The Cervical Cap: Effectiveness, Safety and Acceptability as a Barrier Contraceptive." *The Mount Sinai Journal of Medicine* 53 (4), Apr. 1986.

Lehfeldt, Hans. "Cervical Cap." In *Manual of Family Planning and Contraceptive Practice*. Mary Steichen Calderone, ed. Baltimore: The Williams & Wilkins Co., 1970.

———. "The First Five Years of Contraceptive Service in a Municipal Hospital." *American Journal of Obstetrics and Gynecology* 93 (5), Nov. 1, 1965.

——— and Irving Sivin. "Use Effectiveness of the Prentif Cervical Cap in Private Practice: A Prospective Study." *Contraception* 30 (4), Oct. 1984.

———, Aquiles J. Sobrero and Will Inglis. "Spermicidal Effectiveness of Chemical Contraceptives Used with the Firm Cervical Cap." *American Journal of Obstetrics and Gynecology*, Aug. 1961.

Littman, Karen Joyce. "Contraception: The Cervical Cap: Back to Basics." *Ms.*, Oct. 1980.

Loraine, J. A. "Other Methods of Birth Control." In *Sex and the Population Crisis*. London: William Heinemann, 1970.

Ludwig, Thomas. *Zur Technik der Individuellen Abformung der Portio Vaginalis Uteri.* Inaugural-Dissertation zur Erlangung der Doktorwürde in der Zahnheilkunde an der Ludwig Maximilians-Universität zur München, 1983.

Malasky, Sandra. "Cervical Cap Research Planned for NHFHC." *Womanwise* (New Hampshire Feminist Health Center), Winter 1980.

———— and Susan Jordan. "The Continuing Saga of the Cervical Cap." *Womanwise* (New Hampshire Feminist Health Center), Spring 1981.

Marshall, Joan. "A Reappraisal of Female Barrier Methods of Contraception." *Digest: A Review of Contraceptive Topics,* Nov. 1977.

McBride, G. and C. Arthur. "Customized Cervical Cap." *Journal of Nurse-Midwifery* 25, 1980.

"Mechanical Devices: Procedures for Investigational Device Exemptions." *The Federal Register,* Washington, D.C., Jan. 18, 1979.

Moses, Bessie L. "A Flat Rim Cervical Cap." *Human Fertility* 6, 1944.

Müller, Wolfgang. "Zur Kontrazeption mit Portiokappen." Inaugural-Dissertation zur Erlangung der Doktorwürde in der Zahnheilkunde an der Ludwig Maximilians-Universität zur München, 1983.

National Women's Health Network. "Cervical Cap Update." *Update,* 1981.

"The Newest Contraceptive." *Redbook,* Apr. 1987.

Parker, R. "If the Cap Fits . . ." *Spare Rib,* Mar. 1977.

Patton, Robert. "Cervical Caps." *Cosmopolitan,* June 1981.

Peel, John and Malcolm Potts. "Diaphragms and Caps." *Textbook of Contraceptive Practice.* Cambridge: The University Press, 1969.

Prupes, Karen. "Custom Cervical Cap Reentering Clinical Trials." *Journal of the American Medical Association* 250 (15), Oct. 21, 1983.

Pust, Walter. "Discussion of Mechanical Occlusive Methods." In Sanger and Stone.

Sanger, Margaret. *Birth Control Through the Ages: A Chronological History of the Birth Control Movement from Ancient to Modern Times.* New York: Planned Parenthood Federation of America, 1940.

————. "Family Limitation." 5th ed. Privately printed, 1916.

————. *My Fight for Birth Control*. Elmsford, N.Y.: Maxwell Reprint Co., 1969.

———— and Hannah M. Stone. *The Practice of Contraception*. Baltimore: The Williams & Wilkins Co., 1931.

Sauer, L. "Cervical Cap: A Contraceptive Emerges as Attractive Option." *The New York Times*, Aug. 26, 1980.

Schmid-Tannwald, Ingolf, E. Graf and W. Beitelschmidt. "Individuelle Portioabdrücke beim Menschen. Erste Klinische Ergebnisse." *Mitteilungen der Gesellschaft fur Praktische Sexualmedizin* 4 (4), May 1984.

Schofield, Betty E. "The Calgary Cervical Cap Study." Proceedings of the Canadian Committee for Fertility Research. Conference held at Hotel La Sapiniere, Val David, Quebec, Canada, Nov. 24–25, 1983.

Seaman, Barbara and Gideon Seaman. *Women and the Crisis in Sex Hormones*. New York: Rawson Associates Publishers, 1977 (cloth). New York: Bantam Books, 1978 (paper).

Sein, Muang. "Flexible Plastic Contraceptive Caps: An Ideal Contraceptive for Developing Countries." Unpublished, 1975.

Sherris, Jacqueline D., Sidney H. Moore and Gordon Fox. "New Developments in Vaginal Contraception." *Population Reports*, Series H (7), Jan.–Feb. 1984.

Smith, Grace Geyer. "The Use of Cervical Caps at the University of California/Berkeley." *Journal of the American College Health Association* 29 (2), Oct. 1980.

————. "The Use of Cervical Caps at the University of California/Berkeley: A Survey." *Contraception* 30 (2), Aug. 1984.

Smith, M. and P. Blais. "Preliminary Findings on Used Cervical Caps." *Contraception* 29 (6), June 1984.

Smith, May. "Newer Barrier Contraceptive: The Cervical Cap." *Medical Aspects of Human Sexuality* 19 (10), Oct. 1985.

Stim, Edward M. "The Nonspermicide Fit-free Diaphragm." *Advances in Planned Parenthood* 15 (3), 1980.

Stone, Hannah M. "Occlusive Methods of Contraception." *Journal of Contraception* 2, 1937.

Stone, Hannah M. and Abraham Stone. *The Marriage Manual*. Rev. ed. by Gloria Stone Aitkin and A. J. Sobrero. New York: Simon & Schuster, 1968.

Stopes, Marie Carmichael. *Birth Control Today*. London: The Hogarth Press, 1957.

———. *Contraception*. London: John Bale, Sons and Danielsson, 1923.

———. *The History of Birth Control*. London: G. P. Putnam, 1931.

Tatum, Howard J. and Elizabeth B. Connell-Tatum. "Barrier Contraception: A Comprehensive Overview." *Fertility and Sterility* 36 (1), July 1981.

Tietze, Christopher, Hans Lehfeldt and H. George Liebmann. "The Effectiveness of the Cervical Cap as a Contraceptive Method." *American Journal of Obstetrics and Gynecology* 66 (4), Oct. 1953.

Weisman, Stephanie. "Taking the Profits Out of Birth Control: The Cervical Cap May Be Safer, Too." *The Progressive* 44 (9), Sept. 1980.

Wham, Dashiel. "The Perfect Birth Control and Why You Can't Buy it." *Seattle Weekly*, Jan. 10, 1985. Reprinted in *NFPRHA News* 4 (4), Summer 1985.

Wilde, Friederich A. *Das weibliche Gebärunvermögen*. Berlin, 1838.

Willis, Judith. "Cervical Caps: The Perfect, Untested Contraceptive." *FDA Consumer*, Apr. 1981.

Willis, Mary Sherman. "Cervical Caps: Old, Yet Too New." *Science News*, Dec. 22, 1979.

Wortman, Judith. "The Diaphragm and Other Intravaginal Barriers: A Review." *Population Reports*, Series H (4), Jan. 1976.

Wright, Helena. *Contraceptive Technique*. London: J. and A. Churchill, 1968.

———. "Indications for Use of the Dumas and Pro-Race Cervical Caps." In Sanger and Stone.

Yarros, Rachelle S. "Experience with the Cervical Pessary." In Sanger and Stone.

Zodhiates, Kathryn Porterfield, Richard I. Feinbloom and Stanley E. Sagov. "Contraceptive Use of Cervical Caps." Letter. *New England Journal of Medicine* 304 (15), 1981.

INDEX

Sponge, contraceptive, 6, 8, 14, 88, 104, 119
  survey of, 126–29
Spontaneity, sex and, 91–96, 121
Stein, Linda, 68, 173
Sterilization, 6, 119, 140–43
Stim, Edward, 123, 173
Stone, Hannah, 22–23n
Stopes, Marie, x, 16, 18–19, 21, 174
Stubblefield, Philip, 25
Surgical Instrument Research Laboratory, 20

Teenagers, birth control and, 10, 97–101
Test cap, 174–75
Thogersen, Lynn, 173
Tietze, Christopher, 21, 68, 160–61, 164, 177
Today™ contraceptive sponge. *See* Sponge, contraceptive
Toxic Shock Syndrome (TSS), 8, 67, 88–89, 124, 127
Training
  of cap users, 49–50
  of practitioners, 52–53

United States, cervical cap development in, 14–15, 20–21
Urethral sponge, 63, 92, 94
Users
  confidence of, 50, 52, 73
  description of, 6–7
  discomfort of, 75–76, 94
  failures of, 106–7

profile of ideal, 109
training of, 49–50
Uterus
  prolapsed, 90
  sexual response and, 47

Vacuum aspiration, 163–64
Vagina
  back of, 62
  infections of, 84–85, 90
Vasectomy, 119, 144–46
Vermont Feminist Health Center, 48
Victorian England, cervical cap in, 7, 15–16, 22
Vimule cap, 28–30, 85, 170, 174, 182

Ware Company, x
Washington Women's Self-Help (WWSH), 39, 171, 172
Watkins, P. P. W., 29–30, 34
Watkins, Richard N., 69n
Wheeler, Robert, 116–17
Whipple, Beverly, 91, 92, 175
Wilde, Friedrich A., x, 14, 178
Withdrawal (coitus interruptus), 159–62
Womancap, 5
Women and the Crisis in Sex Hormones (Seaman and Seaman), 1, 24–25, 94
Women's Health Service of Colorado Springs, 42
Wright, Helena, 19

Yarros, Rachelle S., 20
Yin,Lillian, 34, 35